ATKINS DIET
FOOD LIST FOR
EPILEPSY

Easy ways to make delicious recipes for managing epilepsy and seizures, shed weight, and treat other disorders naturally through modified Atkins.

Dr. Emily Thompson

Copyright © 2023 by **Dr. Emily Thompson**

All rights reserved. No part of this book may be used or reproduced in any form whatsoever without written permission except in the case of brief quotations in critical articles or reviews.

Printed in the United States of America.
First Edition: Movember, 2023.

ABOUT THE AUTHOR: DR. EMILY THOMPSON

Dr. Emily Thompson is a distinguished medical professional with a passion for improving the lives of individuals affected by epilepsy through the application of dietary therapies. With over two decades of experience in the field of neurology and dietary interventions, she has become a leading expert in the use of the Modified Atkins Diet for managing epilepsy.

Dr. Thompson's journey into the world of epilepsy and nutrition began during her early medical career when she witnessed the transformative effects of dietary therapy on her patients. Her commitment to seeking innovative solutions for epilepsy management led her to delve deep into the research and practice of therapeutic diets, particularly the Modified Atkins Diet.

Throughout her career, Dr. Thompson has been a tireless advocate for individuals with epilepsy and their families. She has conducted numerous clinical trials, published groundbreaking research, and delivered lectures at international conferences, sharing her wealth of knowledge on dietary therapies.

In addition to her clinical work and research, Dr. Thompson is a dedicated educator, always eager to impart her expertise to the next generation of medical professionals. She has mentored and trained countless physicians, dietitians, and healthcare providers in the intricacies of the Modified Atkins Diet and its applications in epilepsy management.

Dr. Thompson's commitment to patient care goes beyond the clinic. She is known for her compassionate and personalized approach, tailoring treatment plans to suit each patient's unique needs and circumstances. Her holistic view of health underscores the importance of not only managing seizures but also enhancing the overall well-being of her patients.

As an author, Dr. Thompson seeks to make her extensive knowledge and experience accessible to a wider audience. Her upcoming book, "The Modified Atkins Diet for Epilepsy: A Comprehensive Guide," reflects her dedication to empowering individuals and families with practical, evidence-based guidance on using the diet as a tool for improved epilepsy management.

When she's not immersed in the world of neurology and dietary therapies, Dr. Thompson finds solace in the outdoors, where she enjoys hiking, gardening, and unwinding with a good book. Her diverse interests and deep-rooted commitment to her patients make her a respected figure in the field of epilepsy management and dietary therapies.

Dr. Emily Thompson's unwavering dedication to advancing the understanding and implementation of the Modified Atkins Diet in epilepsy management continues to inspire her colleagues, patients, and readers alike. Her work embodies a fusion of medical expertise, scientific inquiry, and genuine compassion, aimed at improving the lives of those affected by epilepsy.

TABLE OF CONTENT

About the Author: Dr. Emily Thompson, MD 3

Introduction: Discovering the Modified Atkins Diet for Health and Epilepsy Management 1

UNDERSTANDING THE MODIFIED ATKINS DIET 3
The Basics of the Atkins Diet 3
Four Phases: 3
a. Induction Phase: 3
b. Balancing Phase (OWL - Ongoing Weight Loss): 3
c. Pre-Maintenance Phase: 4
d. Maintenance Phase: 4
Carbohydrate Restriction: 4
Focus on Protein and Fats: 4

How the Modified Atkins Diet Differs 7

Carbohydrate Intake: 7
Ketosis: 7
Medical Use: 8
Simplicity: 8
Scientific Support: 9

Who Can Benefit from This Diet 10

Epilepsy Patients: 10
Seizure Disorders: 10
Weight Management: 11
Metabolic Conditions: 11
Neurological Conditions: 11
Polycystic Ovary Syndrome (PCOS): 11
Type 2 Diabetes: 12
Cardiovascular Health: 12

Neuropsychiatric Conditions: 12
The Science Behind Epilepsy and Diet 14
Exploring The Relationship Between Diet and Epilepsy 14
Historical Perspective: 14
Ketosis and Seizure Control: 15
The Modified Atkins Diet (MAD): 15
Mechanisms of Action: 15
Patient Selection: 15
Challenges and Considerations: 16
Evolving Research: 16
Mechanisms of Action 18
Ketosis and Altered Brain Metabolism: 18
GABAergic and Glutamatergic Effects: 18
Ion Channel and Neuronal Membrane Stability: 19
Anti-Inflammatory and Antioxidant Effects: 19
Metabolic Competition and Energy Availability: 19
Weight Loss and Hormonal Effects (MAD): 20
Research and Clinical Studies 21
Early Research on the Ketogenic Diet: 21
Modern Clinical Trials: 21
Efficacy in Drug-Resistant Epilepsy: 22
Impact on Quality of Life: 22
Mechanisms of Action: 22
Safety and Tolerability: 23
Applications Beyond Epilepsy: 23
Long-Term Effects and Maintenance: 23
Patient Profiles and Individualized Treatment: 23
Meta-Analyses and Systematic Reviews: 24

Getting Started **25**

Preparing Mentally and Emotionally **25**

Set Clear Goals: 25
Educate Yourself: 25
Seek Professional Guidance: 25
Embrace Change Gradually: 26
Visualize Success: 26
Develop a Support System: 26
Manage Expectations: 26
Practice Self-Compassion: 26
Focus on the Positive: 27
Cultivate Resilience: 27
Embrace a Growth Mindset: 27
Practice Mindfulness: 27
Stay Informed: 27
Celebrate Achievements: 28
Stay Flexible: 28

Consultation with Healthcare Professionals **29**

Primary Care Physician: 29
Specialists: 29
Dietitian or Nutritionist: 30
Mental Health Professionals: 30
Allied Health Professionals: 30
Honest Communication: 31
Ask Questions: 31
Follow Recommendations: 31
Regular Check-Ins: 31
Second Opinions: 32

Patient Advocacy: 32
Setting Realistic Goals **33**

Be Specific: 33
Make Your Goals Measurable: 33
Set Achievable Goals: 33
Relevance Matters: 34
Time-Bound Goals: 34
Break It Down: 34
Account for Challenges: 34
Be Flexible: 34
Seek Professional Guidance: 35
Track Your Progress: 35
Celebrate Achievements: 35
Stay Patient: 35
Avoid Perfectionism: 35
Visualize Success: 36
Stay Accountable: 36
Regularly Review Your Goals: 36

Phases of the Modified Atkins Diet **37**

Gradual Carb Reintroduction **37**

Phased Approach: 37
Adding Carbohydrates: 37
Monitoring Impact: 37
Finding Your Threshold: 38
Individualized Approach: 38
Healthy Choices: 38
Balancing Macros: 38
Sustainability: 39

Step-by-Step Phases: Building a Foundation 40

Step 1: Clarify Your Vision 40
Step 2: Identify Your Values 40
Step 3: Set Specific Goals 40
Step 4: Develop a Plan 40
Step 5: Gather Resources 41
Step 6: Acquire Knowledge and Skills 41
Step 7: Take Action 41
Step 8: Monitor Progress 41
Step 9: Adapt and Learn 42
Step 10: Build a Support Network 42
Step 11: Prioritize Self-Care 42
Step 12: Persevere Through Challenges 42
Step 13: Review and Reflect 42
Step 14: Celebrate Milestones 43
Step 15: Share Your Success 43

Transitioning Between Phases 44

Assess and Reflect: 44
Goal Setting: 44
Planning and Preparation: 44
Timelines and Milestones: 45
Resource Allocation: 45
Communication: 45
Adaptability: 45
Seek Guidance and Support: If 45
Maintain a Positive Mindset: 46
Continuous Learning: 46
Evaluate and Adjust: 46

Celebrate Achievements: 46

Crafting Your Shopping Lists **47**

Fresh Foods and Pantry Staples **47**

1. Fresh Foods: 47
2. Pantry Staples: 48

Navigating the Grocery Store **50**

1. Make a Shopping List: 50
2. Eat Before You Go: 50
3. Stick to the Perimeter: 50
4. Read Labels: 50
5. Compare Prices: 51
6. Buy in Bulk (When Appropriate): 51
7. Choose Fresh Produce Wisely: 51
8. Be Mindful of Sales and Specials: 51
9. Limit Processed Foods: 51
10. Consider Frozen and Canned Varieties: 52
11. Check for Store Brands: 52
12. Stay Hydrated: 52
13. Avoid Impulse Buys: 52
14. Bring Your Own Bags: 52
15. Practice Safe Food Handling: 52
16. Be Patient: 53

Shopping for Success **54**

Setting Clear Goals and Objectives: 54
Budgeting and Financial Responsibility: 54
Distinguishing Needs from Wants: 55
Informed Decision-Making: 55
Organized Shopping: 55

Value and Quality: 55
Ethical and Sustainable Choices: 56
Supporting Local and Small Businesses: 56
Minimalism and Decluttering: 56
Gratitude and Contentment: 57

Delicious Recipes for Every Phase 58

Breakfast 58

1. Avocado and Bacon Breakfast Bowl 58
2. Spinach and Feta Omelette 59
3. Keto Chia Pudding 60
4. Smoked Salmon and Cream Cheese Roll-Ups 61
5. Greek Yogurt Parfait 62
6. Zucchini and Cheese Frittata 63
7. Sausage and Egg Breakfast Casserole 64
8. Peanut Butter and Chocolate Smoothie 65
9. Tomato and Basil Scrambled Eggs 66
10. Coconut and Berry Chia Bowl 67

Lunch: 69

Phase 1: Initial Induction Phase (Classic MAD) 69
1. Avocado and Chicken Salad 69
Phase 2: Ongoing Weight Loss (Classic MAD) 70
2. Spinach and Bacon Quiche 70
Phase 3: Pre-Maintenance and Maintenance (Classic MAD) 71
3. Turkey and Avocado Lettuce Wraps 71
Phase 4: Gradual Transition (Classic MAD) 72
4. Cauliflower Fried Rice 72
Phase 5: Maintenance (Modified MAD) 74

5. Greek Salad with Grilled Chicken 74

Phase 1: Initial Induction Phase (Classic MAD) 75

6. Tuna Salad Lettuce Wraps 75

Phase 2: Ongoing Weight Loss (Classic MAD) 76

7. Broccoli and Cheddar Soup 76

Phase 3: Pre-Maintenance and Maintenance (Classic MAD) 77

8. Egg Salad Stuffed Bell Peppers 77

Phase 4: Gradual Transition (Classic MAD) 78

9. Grilled Shrimp and Asparagus 78

Phase 5: Maintenance (Modified MAD) 79

10. Caprese Salad with Grilled Chicken 79

Dinners 81

Phase 1: Initial Induction Phase (Classic MAD) 81

1. Lemon Garlic Butter Shrimp 81

Phase 2: Ongoing Weight Loss (Classic MAD) 82

2. Cauliflower Alfredo with Grilled Chicken 82

Phase 3: Pre-Maintenance and Maintenance (Classic MAD) 83

3. Beef and Broccoli Stir-Fry 83

Phase 4: Gradual Transition (Classic MAD) 84

4. Spaghetti Squash with Pesto and Grilled Chicken 84

Phase 5: Maintenance (Modified MAD) 85

5. Grilled Salmon with Asparagus 85

Phase 1: Initial Induction Phase (Classic MAD) 86

6. Beef and Cabbage Stir-Fry 86

Phase 2: Ongoing Weight Loss (Classic MAD) 87

7. Creamy Garlic Parmesan Zoodles with Chicken 87

Phase 3: Pre-Maintenance and Maintenance (Classic MAD) 88

8. Sausage and Spinach Stuffed Mushrooms 88

Phase 4: Gradual Transition (Classic MAD) 90

9. Turkey and Avocado Lettuce Wraps..................................90

Phase 5: Maintenance (Modified MAD) 91

10. Grilled Pork Chops with Broccoli 91

Snacks..93

Phase 1: Initial Induction Phase (Classic Mad)....................93

1. Cucumber and Cream Cheese Bites................................93

Phase 2: Ongoing Weight Loss (Classic Mad).....................94

2. Bacon-Wrapped Asparagus Spears 94

Phase 3: Pre-Maintenance and Maintenance (Classic Mad)..95

3. Deviled Eggs 95

Phase 4: Gradual Transition (Classic Mad)..........................96

4. Guacamole with Veggie Sticks..96

Phase 5: Maintenance (Modified MAD................................97

5. Greek Yogurt Parfait 97

Phase 1: Initial Induction Phase (Classic Mad)....................98

6. Cheese and Pepperoni Slices 98

Phase 2: Ongoing Weight Loss (Classic Mad).....................99

7. Avocado Slices with Smoked Salmon 99

Phase 3: Pre-Maintenance and Maintenance (Classic Mad)...100

8. Tuna Cucumber Boats...100

Phase 4: Gradual Transition (Classic Mad)........................101

9. Mozzarella and Tomato Skewers 101
Phase 5: Maintenance (Modified MAD) 102

10. Chocolate Avocado Mousse 102
DESSERTS 104

Phase 1: Initial Induction Phase (Classic MAD) 104

1. Chocolate Avocado Pudding 104
Phase 2: Ongoing Weight Loss (Classic MAD) 105

2. Berry Parfait 105
Phase 3: Pre-Maintenance and Maintenance (Classic MAD) 106

3. Chia Seed Pudding 106
Phase 4: Gradual Transition (Classic MAD) 108

4. Avocado Chocolate Mousse 108
Phase 5: Maintenance (Modified MAD) 109

5. Lemon Cheesecake Fat Bombs 109
Phase 1: Initial Induction Phase (Classic MAD) 110

6. Peanut Butter Chocolate Fat Bombs 110
Phase 2: Ongoing Weight Loss (Classic MAD) 111

7. Vanilla Almond Chia Pudding 111
Phase 3: Pre-Maintenance and Maintenance (Classic MAD) 112

8. Chocolate Covered Strawberries 112
Phase 4: Gradual Transition (Classic MAD) 113

9. Raspberry Almond Fat Bombs 113
Phase 5: Maintenance (Modified MAD) 114

10. Berries and Cream 114

Meal Planning Tips 116
    Understand Your Dietary Phase: 116
    Consult a Dietitian: 116
    Balanced Macronutrients: 116
    Portion Control: 116
    Meal Timing: 117
    Prep and Plan Ahead: 117
    Choose Whole Foods: 117
    Read Labels: 117
    Limit Processed Foods: 117
    Include Fiber: 118
    Stay Hydrated: 118
    Track Your Intake: 118
    Experiment with Recipes: 118
    Plan for Social Situations: 118
    Listen to Your Body: 118
    Be Patient and Persistent: 119

FOOD LIST FOR EPILEPSY 120

A One-Week Meal Plan 122
    Day 1: 122
    Day 2: 122
    Day 3: 123
    Day 4: 123
    Day 5: 123
    Day 6: 124
    Day 7: 124

Convenience Options 125

Low-Cook and No-Cook Solutions 125

Low-Cook Solutions: 125
No-Cook Solutions: 126

Grab-and-Go Foods **128**

1. Nuts and Seeds: 128
2. Hard-Boiled Eggs: 128
3. Cheese Sticks or Slices: 128
4. Deli Meats: 128
5. Canned Tuna or Salmon: 128
6. Avocado Slices: 129
7. Low-Carb Protein Bars: 129
8. Greek Yogurt Cups: 129
9. Beef Jerky: 129
10. Vegetable Sticks: 129
11. Low-Carb Wraps: 129
12. Pre-Made Salads: 129
13. Keto Smoothies: 130
14. Mini Frittatas: 130
15. Sugar-Free Jello Cups: 130

Balancing Convenience with Nutritional Value **131**

1. Prep in Advance: 131
2. Choose Convenient Low-Carb Options: 131
3. Read Labels Carefully: 131
4. Frozen Low-Carb Meals: 131
5. Keep Healthy Snacks on Hand: 131
6. Batch Cooking: 132
7. Meal Replacement Shakes: 132
8. Plan Your Meals: 132
9. Incorporate Convenience Veggies: 132

10. Healthy Convenience Stores: 132
11. Online Shopping: 132
12. Balance with Fresh Foods: 132
13. Limit Processed Convenience Foods: 133
14. Drink Water: 133
15. Consult a Dietitian: 133

Digital Tools and Apps 134

Simplifying Meal Planning 134

1. Set Clear Objectives: 134
2. Understand Your Dietary Phase: 134
3. Create a Go-To List: 134
4. Plan Weekly Menus: 134
5. Batch Cooking: 134
6. Use a Template: 135
7. Rotate Favorite Recipes: 135
8. Simple Meal Components: 135
9. Prep Ingredients: 135
10. Make a Shopping List: 135
11. Explore Convenience Foods: 135
12. Utilize Leftovers: 135
13. Keep It Simple: 136
14. Consult a Dietitian: 136
15. Stay Organized: 136
16. Flexibility: 136

Tracking Your Progress 137

1. Keep a Food Diary: 137
2. Weigh and Measure: 137
3. Monitor Blood Sugar Levels: 137

4.	Record Non-Scale Victories:	137
5.	Use Before and After Photos:	137
6.	Keep a Symptom Journal:	138
7.	Set Clear Goals:	138
8.	Regular Check-Ins:	138
9.	Track Exercise:	138
10.	Assess Mental Health:	138
11.	Create a Progress Chart:	138
12.	Celebrate Milestones:	138
13.	Share Your Progress:	139
14.	Be Patient:	139
15.	Adapt and Adjust:	139
16.	Listen to Your Body:	139

Incorporating Technology into Your Journey 140

1.	Meal Tracking Apps:	140
2.	Recipe Websites and Apps:	140
3.	Fitness Trackers:	140
4.	Blood Sugar Monitors:	140
5.	Smart Kitchen Appliances:	140
6.	Online Support Communities:	141
7.	Telehealth Services:	141
8.	Wearable Fitness Devices:	141
9.	Smart Scales:	141
10.	Meal Planning and Grocery Apps:	141
11.	Food Barcode Scanners:	141
12.	Educational Websites and Podcasts:	141
13.	Medication and Health Apps:	142
14.	Mindfulness and Stress-Reduction Apps:	142
15.	Health Dashboard Apps:	142

16. Cooking Demonstrations: 142

Success Stories and Testimonials 143

Insights and Inspiration from those who've Walked the Path 143

Lessons from Personal Journeys 146

Sustainable Long-Term Health 149

Beyond Weight Loss: A Holistic Approach 149

Mind, Body, and Spirit 149
The Modified Atkins Diet as a Tool 149
Physical Fitness and Movement 150
Mindfulness and Stress Management 150
Social and Community Connections 151
The Essence of Holistic Wellness 151

Strategies for Maintaining Your Progress 152

Making the Modified Atkins Diet a Lifestyle Choice 155

Conclusion: Your Journey to Improved Health Starts Today 159

INTRODUCTION: DISCOVERING THE MODIFIED ATKINS DIET FOR HEALTH AND EPILEPSY MANAGEMENT

In recent years, there has been a growing interest in dietary approaches to manage various health conditions, and one such approach that has gained attention is the Modified Atkins Diet (MAD). Originally developed as a weight loss diet, the Modified Atkins Diet has shown promise in the management of epilepsy, particularly in drug-resistant cases. This dietary regimen represents a significant departure from traditional antiepileptic medications and offers new hope to individuals seeking alternative ways to manage their condition.

Epilepsy is a neurological disorder characterized by recurrent, unprovoked seizures. While many people with epilepsy successfully control their seizures with medication, a significant proportion continues to experience seizures despite taking multiple antiepileptic drugs. For these individuals, the search for effective treatment options often leads them to explore alternative therapies, and the Modified Atkins Diet is one such option.

The Modified Atkins Diet is a low-carbohydrate, high-fat diet that shares some similarities with the ketogenic diet, which has been used for decades to manage epilepsy. However, the Modified Atkins Diet is more permissive and easier to implement, making it a practical choice for many individuals. This diet encourages the consumption of healthy fats, such as avocados, nuts, and olive oil, while minimizing carbohydrate intake. The idea behind this approach is to shift the body's primary source of energy from carbohydrates to fats, resulting in the production of ketones, which are believed to have a stabilizing effect on brain function and reduce the occurrence of seizures.

This introduction aims to shed light on the Modified Atkins Diet, its origins, and its growing relevance in the field of epilepsy management. As we delve deeper into this dietary strategy, we will explore its principles, scientific evidence, and potential benefits and risks. By understanding the Modified Atkins Diet and its implications, individuals affected by epilepsy and healthcare professionals may find valuable insights into an alternative approach to improving their health and quality of life.

CHAPTER ONE

UNDERSTANDING THE MODIFIED ATKINS DIET

The Basics of the Atkins Diet

The Atkins Diet is a popular low-carbohydrate diet that was first introduced by Dr. Robert C. Atkins in the early 1970s. It gained widespread attention and has since evolved into various versions. The core principles of the Atkins Diet revolve around restricting carbohydrates and promoting the consumption of protein and fats for weight loss and improved overall health. Here are the basics of the Atkins Diet:

Four Phases: The Atkins Diet typically consists of four phases, each with its specific goals and dietary recommendations.

a. Induction Phase: This initial phase is the most restrictive, allowing only 20-25 grams of net carbohydrates per day. Net carbohydrates are calculated by subtracting fiber content from total carbohydrates. The focus is on entering a state of ketosis, where the body burns fat for energy.

b. Balancing Phase (OWL - Ongoing Weight Loss): In this phase, you gradually increase your daily carbohydrate intake while continuing to lose weight. The aim is to find your "Critical Carbohydrate Level for Losing" (CCLL), where you can lose weight while consuming more carbohydrates without gaining it back.

c. Pre-Maintenance Phase: As you approach your weight loss goal, you slow down the rate of weight loss by further increasing your daily carbohydrate intake. This phase prepares you for long-term maintenance.

d. Maintenance Phase: In the maintenance phase, you identify your "Critical Carbohydrate Level for Maintenance" (CCLM), the level at which you can maintain your weight without gaining or losing. You continue to follow a controlled carbohydrate diet to sustain your results.

Carbohydrate Restriction: The foundation of the Atkins Diet is significantly limiting your carbohydrate intake. It's designed to shift the body's primary source of energy from carbohydrates to fats, encouraging a state of ketosis. Foods high in sugar, grains, and starchy vegetables are restricted during the initial phases.

Focus on Protein and Fats: The Atkins Diet emphasizes the consumption of protein and healthy fats, such as avocados, nuts, seeds, and olive oil. These foods provide satiety and help maintain energy levels while keeping carbohydrate intake low.

Food Choices: Allowed foods include meat, poultry, fish, eggs, non-starchy vegetables, and dairy products. Sugary and starchy foods, like bread, pasta, and sugary beverages, are limited or eliminated.

Individualized Approach: The Atkins Diet is flexible and can be tailored to individual needs and preferences. Some variations of the diet accommodate vegetarian or vegan lifestyles.

Potential Benefits: The Atkins Diet may lead to weight loss, improved blood sugar control, and reduced triglyceride levels in some individuals. It can also be an effective tool for those seeking to break free from sugar addiction and unhealthy eating habits.

Criticisms and Considerations: Critics argue that the Atkins Diet can be high in saturated fats and may lack essential nutrients from fruits, whole grains, and legumes. Long-term effects on health are a subject of ongoing research and debate.

Before starting the Atkins Diet or any low-carbohydrate diet, it's advisable to consult with a healthcare professional to ensure it's suitable for your specific health goals and needs. Additionally, maintaining a balanced and nutritious diet is key to long-term health and well-being.

HOW THE MODIFIED ATKINS DIET DIFFERS

The Modified Atkins Diet (MAD) is a variation of the traditional Atkins Diet, with some key differences in its approach and objectives. While both diets share a focus on carbohydrate restriction, there are notable distinctions between the two:

Carbohydrate Intake:

Traditional Atkins Diet: In the induction phase of the Atkins Diet, carbohydrate intake is extremely restricted, often limited to 20-25 grams of net carbohydrates per day. This strict restriction is intended to induce a state of ketosis.

Modified Atkins Diet: The MAD is less restrictive in terms of carbohydrate intake. It allows for a higher daily carbohydrate limit, typically ranging from 10 to 20% of total daily caloric intake, which is roughly 20-50 grams of net carbohydrates per day. This makes it easier to follow and more practical for many individuals.

Ketosis:

Traditional Atkins Diet: The primary goal of the Atkins Diet is to maintain a state of ketosis, where the body relies on fat for energy. Achieving and maintaining ketosis is a central aspect of the diet.

Modified Atkins Diet: While ketosis may occur to some extent in the MAD, it is not the primary focus. The MAD aims to provide a practical and sustainable approach to carbohydrate restriction without strict ketosis requirements.

Medical Use:

Traditional Atkins Diet: Originally designed by Dr. Atkins as a weight loss diet, the Atkins Diet has evolved into various versions, but its primary application remains weight management.

Modified Atkins Diet: The MAD was developed specifically for medical purposes, with a primary focus on the management of drug-resistant epilepsy, particularly in children and adolescents. It has shown promise in reducing the frequency and severity of seizures.

Simplicity:

Traditional Atkins Diet: The Atkins Diet involves multiple phases, including induction, balancing, pre-maintenance, and maintenance phases, which can be complex to navigate.

Modified Atkins Diet: The MAD is simpler and easier to implement. It typically doesn't include distinct phases, making it a more straightforward dietary approach.

Scientific Support:

Traditional Atkins Diet: There is extensive research and literature on the traditional Atkins Diet, primarily related to weight loss and metabolic health.

Modified Atkins Diet: MAD research primarily focuses on its effectiveness in epilepsy management, especially in pediatric populations. It may have a narrower scope in terms of scientific studies.

In summary, the Modified Atkins Diet differs from the traditional Atkins Diet in terms of its carbohydrate intake, the primary goal, its medical application, simplicity, and scientific focus. The MAD is a modified version of the Atkins Diet tailored for specific medical purposes, particularly in the management of epilepsy, and offers a more flexible and practical approach to carbohydrate restriction. Individuals considering the MAD for epilepsy management should do so under the guidance of healthcare professionals familiar with this dietary therapy.

WHO CAN BENEFIT FROM THIS DIET

The Modified Atkins Diet (MAD) is primarily used as a therapeutic dietary approach for individuals with specific medical conditions. While it was originally developed for the management of drug-resistant epilepsy, the diet has shown promise in addressing other health issues. Here's a breakdown of who can potentially benefit from the MAD:

Epilepsy Patients:

- **Drug-Resistant Epilepsy:** The MAD is often prescribed to individuals, particularly children and adolescents, who have epilepsy that does not respond well to traditional antiepileptic medications. It can help reduce the frequency and severity of seizures in some cases.

Seizure Disorders:

- **Other Seizure Disorders:** In addition to epilepsy, the MAD may be considered for individuals with other types of seizure disorders, such as Lennox-Gastaut syndrome or Dravet syndrome.

Weight Management:

- **Weight Loss:** While not its primary purpose, the MAD, like the traditional Atkins Diet, may be adopted by individuals looking to lose weight. It can help control appetite and promote fat loss due to the low carbohydrate and higher fat content.

Metabolic Conditions:

- **Metabolic Syndrome:** The MAD may benefit individuals with metabolic syndrome, as it can help improve insulin sensitivity, lower triglycerides, and enhance blood sugar control.

Neurological Conditions:

- **Neurological Disorders:** Some research suggests that the MAD might have potential applications in the management of certain neurological conditions beyond epilepsy, such as Parkinson's disease or migraine.

Polycystic Ovary Syndrome (PCOS):

- **Hormonal and Reproductive Health:** For individuals with PCOS, a condition marked by insulin resistance, the MAD may help improve insulin sensitivity, manage weight, and regulate hormonal imbalances.

Type 2 Diabetes:

- **Blood Sugar Control:** The MAD could be considered by individuals with type 2 diabetes to help control blood sugar levels, especially when traditional diabetes management strategies have limited success.

Cardiovascular Health:

- **Cardiovascular Risk Factors:** The MAD may benefit individuals at risk of heart disease by improving lipid profiles and promoting a healthier balance of fats in the diet.

Neuropsychiatric Conditions:

- **Neuropsychiatric Disorders:** Some preliminary research suggests that the MAD might have potential applications in the management of conditions like autism spectrum disorders or bipolar disorder, although further studies are needed.

It's important to note that the MAD should be initiated under the guidance of healthcare professionals, especially when used for medical purposes. The diet may not be suitable for everyone, and individualized guidance is essential to ensure that it is used safely and effectively, considering specific health conditions and goals.

CHAPTER TWO

THE SCIENCE BEHIND EPILEPSY AND DIET EXPLORING THE RELATIONSHIP BETWEEN DIET AND EPILEPSY

Epilepsy is a neurological disorder characterized by recurrent and unprovoked seizures, affecting millions of people worldwide. While antiepileptic medications are the standard treatment for most individuals with epilepsy, a growing body of research has unveiled a strong relationship between diet and the management of this condition. In this exploration, we will delve into the evolving understanding of the connection between diet and epilepsy, with a particular focus on dietary therapies like the Modified Atkins Diet and the ketogenic diet.

Historical Perspective:

The link between diet and epilepsy management is not a recent discovery. In the early 20th century, fasting was observed to reduce seizure activity, laying the groundwork for dietary treatments.

The ketogenic diet, a high-fat, low-carbohydrate diet that induces ketosis, was developed in the 1920s as an epilepsy treatment and became a cornerstone of dietary therapy for the condition.

Ketosis and Seizure Control:

Ketosis, a metabolic state where the body predominantly uses fats for energy, has been associated with reduced seizure activity. The mechanism underlying this effect is still not fully understood but is believed to involve changes in brain energy metabolism and neurotransmitter function.

The Modified Atkins Diet (MAD):

The Modified Atkins Diet is a more palatable and flexible version of the ketogenic diet, designed to be easier to follow. It restricts carbohydrates and encourages a higher intake of fats and proteins.

Research has shown that the MAD can be effective in reducing seizures in people with drug-resistant epilepsy, especially in children and adolescents.

Mechanisms of Action:

While the precise mechanisms of how the MAD and ketogenic diet work to control seizures are not fully elucidated, they are thought to involve changes in brain metabolism, increased levels of ketone bodies, and potentially modulation of neurotransmitters and ion channels.

Patient Selection:

Dietary therapies are often considered for individuals with drug-resistant epilepsy who do not respond well to conventional antiepileptic medications.

It's crucial for patients to be assessed by healthcare professionals, including dietitians, to determine their suitability for dietary interventions and to create tailored diet plans.

Challenges and Considerations:

Adhering to a strict dietary regimen can be challenging and may lead to side effects, such as gastrointestinal issues, vitamin and mineral deficiencies, and lipid imbalances.

Continuous medical monitoring is necessary during dietary therapies, and individuals may need to transition back to a regular diet under professional supervision.

Evolving Research:

Ongoing research is exploring the impact of diet on epilepsy management, including potential applications in various types of epilepsy and the long-term effects of dietary therapies.

Dietary therapies are also being investigated in other neurological and neuropsychiatric conditions, broadening their potential impact.

In conclusion, the relationship between diet and epilepsy management is a fascinating and evolving field of study. Dietary therapies like the Modified Atkins Diet and the ketogenic diet offer hope to individuals with drug-resistant epilepsy and other neurological conditions. As our understanding of these therapies deepens, they may become increasingly valuable tools in the arsenal of treatments for epilepsy, ultimately improving the quality of life for those affected by this challenging condition.

MECHANISMS OF ACTION

The mechanisms of action behind the efficacy of dietary therapies like the Modified Atkins Diet (MAD) and the ketogenic diet in managing epilepsy, particularly drug-resistant epilepsy, are not fully understood but have been a subject of research and hypothesis. Here are some of the proposed mechanisms:

Ketosis and Altered Brain Metabolism:

A key feature of both the MAD and the ketogenic diet is the induction of ketosis, a metabolic state in which the body produces and uses ketone bodies for energy instead of carbohydrates.

It is believed that the presence of ketone bodies, such as beta-hydroxybutyrate, acetoacetate, and acetone, may contribute to reduced seizure activity. Ketones serve as an alternative fuel source for the brain, and this metabolic shift may alter the electrical and chemical activity in the brain, making it less prone to seizures.

GABAergic and Glutamatergic Effects:

Some research suggests that ketosis may influence the balance of neurotransmitters in the brain. It is believed that ketones might enhance the activity of the inhibitory neurotransmitter gamma-aminobutyric acid (GABA) while reducing the excitatory neurotransmitter glutamate. This shift in the neurotransmitter balance may help reduce neuronal hyperexcitability, a key factor in seizure generation.

Ion Channel and Neuronal Membrane Stability:

Ketosis might influence ion channels and the stability of neuronal membranes. Some studies propose that ketones could modulate ion channel activity and membrane properties in a way that decreases neuronal excitability and hyperexcitability, potentially reducing the likelihood of seizures.

Anti-Inflammatory and Antioxidant Effects:

Ketones may have anti-inflammatory and antioxidant properties, which could protect brain cells from damage and inflammation associated with seizure activity. Lowering inflammation and oxidative stress in the brain might contribute to seizure control.

Metabolic Competition and Energy Availability:

The reduced availability of glucose (the primary energy source for the brain in a standard diet) and the presence of ketones create metabolic competition in the brain.

In this altered metabolic environment, it is theorized that neurons relying on glucose may become less active while those using ketones as an energy source may become more active, potentially leading to improved brain stability and fewer seizures.

Weight Loss and Hormonal Effects (MAD):

In the case of the Modified Atkins Diet (MAD), which is often used for epilepsy management, weight loss and improvements in hormonal factors related to insulin resistance may contribute to its effectiveness. These effects can be particularly relevant in patients with obesity-related seizures or insulin resistance.

It's important to note that while these mechanisms are proposed, the exact ways in which the MAD, the ketogenic diet, and other dietary therapies work to reduce seizures in epilepsy are still an area of ongoing research. The effectiveness of these diets can vary among individuals, and their application is typically done under the supervision of healthcare professionals to ensure safety and efficacy. Further research is needed to gain a deeper understanding of the precise mechanisms and optimize dietary therapies for epilepsy management.

RESEARCH AND CLINICAL STUDIES

Research and clinical studies play a pivotal role in advancing our understanding of dietary therapies, like the Modified Atkins Diet (MAD) and the ketogenic diet, for the management of epilepsy. These studies provide critical insights into the safety and efficacy of these treatments. Here is an overview of research and clinical studies related to dietary therapies for epilepsy:

Early Research on the Ketogenic Diet:

The ketogenic diet, one of the oldest dietary therapies for epilepsy, has been the subject of research since the early 20th century. Initial studies, often observational in nature, provided evidence of the diet's effectiveness in reducing seizure frequency, particularly in children with drug-resistant epilepsy.

Modern Clinical Trials:

In recent decades, randomized controlled trials (RCTs) have been conducted to assess the efficacy of dietary therapies more rigorously. These trials involve a control group (often receiving a standard treatment or a placebo) and a group following the MAD or ketogenic diet. Such studies help establish the diets' effectiveness compared to other treatments.

Efficacy in Drug-Resistant Epilepsy:

Numerous clinical trials have specifically targeted individuals with drug-resistant epilepsy to evaluate the impact of dietary therapies. Research has demonstrated that a significant percentage of patients experience a reduction in seizure frequency and severity, sometimes achieving seizure freedom.

Impact on Quality of Life:

Research has also assessed the effects of dietary therapies on the quality of life of individuals with epilepsy. Some studies have shown improvements in mood, cognitive function, and overall well-being among those following the MAD or ketogenic diet.

Mechanisms of Action:

Investigative studies have delved into the mechanisms by which dietary therapies influence epilepsy. Research on animal models and cell cultures has explored the effects of ketosis, alterations in neurotransmitter balance, and changes in ion channel activity.

Safety and Tolerability:

Clinical studies have examined the safety and tolerability of dietary therapies. Researchers have investigated potential side effects, nutrient deficiencies, and lipid imbalances, as well as ways to mitigate these issues.

Applications Beyond Epilepsy:

Some clinical research has explored the use of dietary therapies for conditions beyond epilepsy, such as neurodegenerative diseases, autism spectrum disorders, and mood disorders. These studies are often preliminary and focused on understanding the potential broader applications of these diets.

Long-Term Effects and Maintenance:

Long-term studies have assessed the sustainability and potential long-term effects of dietary therapies, including their impact on growth and development in children. Research has also examined the challenges of maintaining these diets over extended periods.

Patient Profiles and Individualized Treatment:

Research has contributed to the identification of patient profiles most likely to benefit from dietary therapies. Understanding which individuals are more likely to respond positively allows for more targeted treatment plans.

Meta-Analyses and Systematic Reviews:

Meta-analyses and systematic reviews combine data from multiple studies to provide a comprehensive overview of the evidence surrounding dietary therapies for epilepsy. These analyses help to draw more robust conclusions.

It's important to note that while research supports the use of dietary therapies for epilepsy management, these approaches may not be suitable for everyone. The decision to pursue dietary therapy should be made in consultation with healthcare professionals who can consider individual circumstances and medical history. As research continues to evolve, it will likely provide further insights into the optimization and customization of dietary treatments for epilepsy and related conditions.

CHAPTER THREE

GETTING STARTED
PREPARING MENTALLY AND EMOTIONALLY

Undertaking any significant change in your life, whether it's adopting a new diet, embarking on a health journey, or facing a medical condition, often requires mental and emotional preparation. Here are some essential steps to help you get mentally and emotionally ready for the road ahead:

Set Clear Goals:

Define your goals and what you hope to achieve. Whether you're starting a new diet or managing a health condition, having clear objectives will provide motivation and direction.

Educate Yourself:

Gather information about your diet or health condition. Understanding the reasons behind your choices empowers you to make informed decisions and feel more in control.

Seek Professional Guidance:

Consult with healthcare professionals, such as doctors, dietitians, or therapists, who can provide expert advice, personalized guidance, and address your concerns.

Embrace Change Gradually:

Major lifestyle changes can be overwhelming. Consider making gradual adjustments to your diet or health routine, allowing your mind and body to adapt at a manageable pace.

Visualize Success:

Imagine what success looks like for you. Visualizing the positive outcomes can boost your motivation and provide a mental image to work towards.

Develop a Support System:

Share your goals and challenges with trusted friends or family members. Having a support system in place can provide emotional support, encouragement, and accountability.

Manage Expectations:

Understand that challenges may arise, and progress may not always be linear. Be prepared for setbacks and learn to view them as opportunities for growth.

Practice Self-Compassion:

Be kind to yourself. Avoid self-criticism and acknowledge that it's okay to have moments of difficulty or moments when you deviate from your plan.

Focus on the Positive:

Concentrate on the benefits of your choices. Remind yourself of the improvements you've already experienced or the progress you've made.

Cultivate Resilience:

Develop resilience by adapting to change, learning from difficulties, and bouncing back from setbacks. Resilience is a valuable skill for facing challenges.

Embrace a Growth Mindset:

Adopt a growth mindset, believing that you can learn and adapt to new situations. This mindset can help you view challenges as opportunities for personal growth.

Practice Mindfulness:

Mindfulness techniques, such as meditation and deep breathing, can help you stay present and reduce anxiety related to change or uncertainty.

Stay Informed:

Keep up with the latest research and developments related to your diet or health condition. Knowledge can empower you and help you make informed choices.

Celebrate Achievements:

Recognize and celebrate your accomplishments, no matter how small. Positive reinforcement can boost your motivation and morale.

Stay Flexible:

Be open to adjusting your approach if needed. What works best may change over time, and flexibility in your mindset can lead to better outcomes.

Remember that preparing mentally and emotionally is an ongoing process. As you navigate the challenges and successes of your diet or health journey, continue to check in with your emotions and adjust your mental approach as needed. With a strong mindset and emotional resilience, you can better cope with change and work towards your health and wellness goals.

CONSULTATION WITH HEALTHCARE PROFESSIONALS

When embarking on a significant health journey, managing a medical condition, or making substantial dietary changes, it's crucial to consult with healthcare professionals. Their expertise and guidance can provide you with the necessary support, ensure your safety, and help you achieve your health and wellness goals. Here are some key considerations for consulting with healthcare professionals:

Primary Care Physician:

Start by consulting your primary care physician or general practitioner. They can provide an overall assessment of your health, identify any pre-existing conditions, and recommend necessary screenings or tests.

Specialists:

If you have a specific medical condition, consider consulting a specialist who has expertise in that area. For example, if you're managing epilepsy and considering dietary therapy, an epileptologist or a neurologist with experience in this field can provide valuable insights.

Dietitian or Nutritionist:

When making dietary changes, especially if you're exploring specialized diets like the Modified Atkins Diet or the ketogenic diet, consult a registered dietitian or nutritionist. They can help you create a balanced and tailored eating plan, address nutritional concerns, and monitor your progress.

Mental Health Professionals:

The mental and emotional aspects of health journeys are significant. If you're struggling with emotional challenges or need support in maintaining mental well-being, consider consulting a psychologist, psychiatrist, or counselor.

Allied Health Professionals:

Depending on your specific needs, other allied health professionals like physical therapists, occupational therapists, or speech therapists may be relevant to your journey. They can offer guidance and therapies that complement your overall care.

Pharmacist:

If you're taking medications, consult with your pharmacist to ensure that any dietary changes do not interact negatively with your medications. They can provide insights into medication management.

Holistic Practitioners:

If you're interested in complementary or alternative therapies, such as herbal remedies or acupuncture, consult with holistic practitioners. However, be sure to communicate these therapies with your medical team to ensure they align with your overall care plan.

Honest Communication:

Be open and honest with your healthcare professionals about your goals, challenges, and any concerns you may have. Transparent communication enables them to provide the most effective guidance.

Ask Questions:

Don't hesitate to ask questions about your condition, treatment options, and any dietary or lifestyle changes you're considering. Knowledge is a powerful tool in managing your health.

Follow Recommendations:

After consulting with healthcare professionals, it's essential to follow their recommendations and treatment plans diligently. Consistency in your care is often key to achieving positive outcomes.

Regular Check-Ins:

Maintain regular check-ins with your healthcare team to track your progress, adjust your treatment plan as needed, and address any emerging issues promptly.

Second Opinions:

In complex medical cases, seeking a second opinion from another qualified healthcare professional can provide valuable insights and peace of mind.

Patient Advocacy:

Consider having an advocate, such as a trusted friend or family member, accompany you to appointments to help ask questions, take notes, and provide emotional support.

Remember that healthcare professionals are there to guide and support you on your journey to better health. Their expertise is an invaluable resource, and collaboration with them can lead to more successful outcomes and improved well-being.

SETTING REALISTIC GOALS

Setting realistic goals is a fundamental step in any health or personal development journey. Realistic goals are achievable and motivating, and they provide a clear roadmap for success. Here are some guidelines to help you set realistic goals:

Be Specific:

Clearly define your goal. Vague or general objectives are challenging to measure and work towards. Instead of saying, "I want to be healthier," specify, "I want to reduce my cholesterol levels."

Make Your Goals Measurable:

Create criteria for tracking your progress. This could involve quantifiable metrics like pounds lost, miles run, or blood pressure readings. Measurable goals allow you to assess your success objectively.

Set Achievable Goals:

Ensure that your goals are realistic and attainable given your current circumstances, resources, and constraints. Setting overly ambitious goals can lead to frustration and discouragement.

Relevance Matters:

Your goals should align with your values and priorities. Ask yourself why a particular goal is essential to you and how it contributes to your well-being or overall objectives.

Time-Bound Goals:

Establish a timeframe for achieving your goals. Whether it's a daily, weekly, or monthly deadline, having a sense of urgency can help keep you motivated and accountable.

Break It Down:

Large goals can be intimidating. Divide them into smaller, manageable tasks or milestones. This makes the process less overwhelming and allows you to celebrate achievements along the way.

Account for Challenges:

Recognize that obstacles and setbacks are part of any journey. Anticipate potential challenges and strategize how you'll overcome them.

Be Flexible:

Life can be unpredictable, and circumstances may change. Be willing to adapt your goals when needed. Flexibility is key to long-term success.

Seek Professional Guidance:

Consult with healthcare professionals, dietitians, or fitness experts when setting health-related goals. They can help you create goals that are safe and attainable.

Track Your Progress:

Keep a record of your progress. This could be a journal, a mobile app, or regular check-ins with a healthcare professional. Tracking helps you stay accountable and motivated.

Celebrate Achievements:

Acknowledge and celebrate your successes, no matter how small. Positive reinforcement can boost motivation and morale.

Stay Patient:

Rome wasn't built in a day, and meaningful change takes time. Be patient with yourself and understand that progress may be gradual.

Avoid Perfectionism:

Striving for perfection can be demotivating. Accept that you'll have moments of imperfection and that it's a natural part of the process.

Visualize Success:

Create a mental image of yourself achieving your goals. Visualization can be a powerful motivator.

Stay Accountable:

Share your goals with a friend, family member, or support group. Accountability to others can help you stay on track.

Regularly Review Your Goals:

Periodically assess your progress and adjust your goals as needed. This reflective process ensures that your objectives remain relevant and achievable.

Setting realistic goals is the foundation of effective personal and health-related progress. By following these guidelines and tailoring your goals to your unique situation, you'll increase your chances of success and enjoy a more fulfilling and sustainable health journey.

CHAPTER FOUR

PHASES OF THE MODIFIED ATKINS DIET GRADUAL CARB REINTRODUCTION

Gradual carb reintroduction is a dietary strategy used in various low-carbohydrate diets, including the Atkins Diet and the Modified Atkins Diet, to transition from the initial phases, which are highly restrictive in terms of carbohydrate intake, to a more balanced and sustainable long-term approach. This process involves slowly reintroducing carbohydrates into the diet to find an individual's tolerance level while still maintaining weight loss or other therapeutic goals. Here's how gradual carb reintroduction typically works:

Phased Approach: As you progress through the initial phases of a low-carb diet, where carb intake is extremely restricted, you eventually reach a point where you've achieved your short-term goals, such as weight loss, and are ready to transition to a more flexible, long-term eating plan.

Adding Carbohydrates: During the gradual carb reintroduction phase, you systematically add more carbohydrates back into your daily diet. This is done in a controlled and structured manner.

Monitoring Impact: It's essential to monitor the impact of these added carbohydrates on your body. You pay attention to factors such as weight changes, energy levels, hunger, and how the carbohydrates affect your overall well-being.

Finding Your Threshold: The goal is to find your personal carbohydrate threshold, often referred to as the "Critical Carbohydrate Level for Losing" (CCLL) in the Atkins Diet. This is the point at which you can consume a moderate amount of carbohydrates without gaining weight or experiencing adverse effects.

Individualized Approach: Carb reintroduction is highly individualized. Some people may find that they can comfortably include a higher number of carbohydrates in their diet, while others may need to remain on a relatively low-carb plan to maintain their goals.

Healthy Choices: As you reintroduce carbohydrates, it's essential to focus on healthy, complex carbohydrates, such as whole grains, fruits, and vegetables, rather than sugary or processed foods. This promotes balanced nutrition.

Balancing Macros: While you increase your carb intake, you also continue to balance your macronutrients (carbohydrates, proteins, and fats) to meet your specific dietary needs and health objectives.

Sustainability: The aim of gradual carb reintroduction is to make the dietary transition more sustainable for the long term. This approach acknowledges that strict carb restriction may not be maintainable indefinitely and that a more balanced and flexible approach can promote continued success.

It's important to note that the pace and extent of carb reintroduction can vary from person to person, and some individuals may need to remain on a relatively low-carb diet to manage specific health conditions or personal preferences. As with any dietary changes, consulting with a healthcare professional or registered dietitian is advisable, as they can provide personalized guidance and ensure that your dietary choices align with your health goals and requirements.

STEP-BY-STEP PHASES: BUILDING A FOUNDATION

Here are the step-by-step phases for building a strong foundation:

Step 1: Clarify Your Vision

Begin by clearly defining your vision or the purpose of what you're building. What is the ultimate goal or outcome you want to achieve? Having a clear vision provides direction and motivation.

Step 2: Identify Your Values

Determine your core values and principles that will guide your actions and decisions throughout the foundation-building process. This helps ensure that your foundation aligns with your beliefs and ethics.

Step 3: Set Specific Goals

Break down your vision into specific, measurable, and time-bound goals. These smaller objectives make your vision more achievable and allow you to track progress.

Step 4: Develop a Plan

Create a detailed plan or roadmap outlining the steps and actions needed to reach your goals. This plan should include timelines, resources required, and potential obstacles.

Step 5: Gather Resources

Identify and secure the resources necessary to execute your plan. Resources may include funding, equipment, expertise, and personnel.

Step 6: Acquire Knowledge and Skills

Invest in acquiring the knowledge and skills needed to execute your plan effectively. Education and training are essential for building a strong foundation.

Step 7: Take Action

Begin implementing your plan and take the necessary actions to move closer to your goals. Consistent and focused effort is key to building a solid foundation.

Step 8: Monitor Progress

Regularly assess your progress by measuring your achievements against your goals. This helps you stay on track and make adjustments as needed.

Step 9: Adapt and Learn

Be open to adaptation and learning from your experiences. Embrace change and use setbacks as opportunities for growth and improvement.

Step 10: Build a Support Network

Surround yourself with a supportive network of people who can provide guidance, encouragement, and feedback. Collaboration and mentorship can be invaluable.

Step 11: Prioritize Self-Care

Don't neglect your physical and mental well-being. Taking care of yourself ensures that you have the energy and resilience to build a strong foundation.

Step 12: Persevere Through Challenges

Expect and embrace challenges as part of the journey. Maintain a strong sense of determination and resilience when faced with obstacles.

Step 13: Review and Reflect

Periodically review your goals, strategies, and progress. Reflect on what's working well and what needs improvement.

Step 14: Celebrate Milestones

Celebrate your achievements, no matter how small. Acknowledging your progress boosts motivation and provides a sense of accomplishment.

Step 15: Share Your Success

Share your experiences and knowledge with others. Your journey can inspire and help others as they work on building their own foundations.

Building a strong foundation is a dynamic and ongoing process. It requires a combination of careful planning, consistent effort, self-awareness, adaptability, and the support of others. Whether you're building a project, a business, or your personal development, these steps can guide you toward success.

TRANSITIONING BETWEEN PHASES

Transitioning between phases is a crucial aspect of any process, ensuring a smooth and effective progression. Whether you're moving from one stage of a project to the next, transitioning from one life milestone to another, or making changes in your personal development journey, these transitions require careful planning and execution. Here are some key considerations and strategies for successfully navigating transitions:

Assess and Reflect: Before moving from one phase to the next, take the time to assess where you currently stand. Reflect on your achievements, challenges, and lessons learned in the previous phase. This self-awareness will help you set the right course for the transition.

Goal Setting: Clearly define your goals for the upcoming phase. What do you want to achieve? What are your priorities and objectives? Setting specific, measurable, and realistic goals provides a roadmap for your transition.

Planning and Preparation: Create a detailed plan that outlines the steps and actions required for a smooth transition. Identify potential obstacles and develop strategies to overcome them. Adequate preparation can alleviate stress and uncertainty during the changeover.

Timelines and Milestones: Establish timelines and milestones to track your progress during the transition. This allows you to measure your success and adjust your approach if needed. Timelines provide a sense of structure and accountability.

Resource Allocation: Determine the resources, both tangible and intangible, needed for the next phase. This could include time, finances, knowledge, and support from others. Ensure you have access to these resources as you move forward.

Communication: Effective communication is essential, whether you're transitioning in a professional context or in personal life. Keep stakeholders informed and involved, share your plans, and address any concerns or questions that may arise.

Adaptability: Be prepared to adapt to unforeseen changes and challenges. Flexibility is key to managing transitions, as unexpected circumstances can arise at any time.

Seek Guidance and Support: If you're uncertain about the transition or facing a complex phase change, don't hesitate to seek guidance from mentors, peers, or experts. They can provide valuable insights and advice.

Maintain a Positive Mindset: A positive attitude can greatly influence the success of your transition. Embrace change as an opportunity for growth and development. Focus on the benefits and possibilities that lie ahead.

Continuous Learning: Continuously acquire knowledge and skills relevant to the next phase. Learning is a powerful tool for adapting and thriving in new situations.

Evaluate and Adjust: Regularly evaluate your progress and adjust as needed. If you encounter obstacles or find that your goals have evolved, don't be afraid to modify your approach.

Celebrate Achievements: Celebrate your achievements and milestones along the way. Recognizing your progress and successes will boost your motivation and morale.

Successful transitioning requires a combination of thoughtful planning, adaptability, and perseverance. By following these strategies and remaining focused on your goals, you can navigate changes with confidence and achieve your desired outcomes.

CHAPTER FIVE

CRAFTING YOUR SHOPPING LISTS
FRESH FOODS AND PANTRY STAPLES

"Fresh Foods and Pantry Staples" are two fundamental categories of items commonly found in kitchens, each serving distinct roles in meal preparation and daily nutrition. Let's delve into these categories:

1. Fresh Foods:

Fresh foods encompass perishable items that are typically bought and consumed within a short timeframe. These items are prized for their natural flavors and nutritional value. Common fresh foods include:

Fruits: Such as apples, bananas, berries, citrus fruits, and more, providing essential vitamins, fiber, and natural sugars.

Vegetables: Including leafy greens, tomatoes, carrots, and broccoli, which offer vitamins, minerals, and dietary fiber.

Meat and Seafood: Such as chicken, beef, fish, and shellfish, serving as primary sources of protein.

Dairy Products: Like milk, yogurt, and cheese, rich in calcium and protein.

Eggs: A versatile source of protein and essential nutrients.

Bakery Items: Such as bread, pastries, and tortillas, providing carbohydrates for energy.

Herbs and Spices: Fresh herbs and dried spices that enhance flavor in cooking.

Fresh foods are integral to a balanced and nutritious diet, often associated with healthy eating habits due to their nutrient-rich profiles and natural flavors.

2. Pantry Staples:

Pantry staples are non-perishable items with a longer shelf life, usually stored in the pantry, cupboard, or another cool, dry area. These items serve as the foundation for creating a wide range of meals and include:

Canned Goods: Such as beans, tomatoes, and vegetables, offering convenience and extending the availability of specific ingredients.

Grains and Pasta: This category encompasses rice, pasta, oats, and various types of grains, serving as important sources of carbohydrates.

Flour and Baking Ingredients: Flour, sugar, baking powder, and other essentials used in baking and cooking.

Cooking Oils and Vinegars: Olive oil, vegetable oil, and various vinegars employed in various recipes.

Cereals and Breakfast Foods: Cereals, granola, and oatmeal, commonly chosen for breakfast.

Canned Soups and Broths: These serve as a base for soups, stews, and sauces.

Spices and Seasonings: A range of spices, herbs, and seasonings that enhance the flavor of dishes.

Nuts and Seeds: Such as almonds, peanuts, and chia seeds, serving as excellent sources of healthy fats and protein.

Condiments: Including ketchup, mustard, mayonnaise, and salad dressings.

Pantry staples are essential for meal planning, particularly when access to fresh foods is limited. They contribute to the convenience and versatility of cooking, as they can be combined with fresh ingredients to create a wide variety of dishes.

Balancing fresh foods and pantry staples is key to maintaining a well-rounded and flexible kitchen, ensuring that you have both the basics and fresh ingredients on hand to prepare a variety of wholesome meals.

NAVIGATING THE GROCERY STORE

Navigating the grocery store efficiently and effectively is a valuable skill for making healthy, budget-conscious food choices. Here are some tips and strategies to help you navigate the grocery store with confidence:

1. Make a Shopping List:

Plan your meals for the week and create a detailed shopping list. Organize the list by categories, such as fruits, vegetables, dairy, etc., to match the store's layout.

2. Eat Before You Go:

Shopping on an empty stomach can lead to impulse purchases of unhealthy snacks and items you don't need. Eat a meal or snack before heading to the store.

3. Stick to the Perimeter:

The perimeter of the store typically contains fresh produce, meat, dairy, and bread. This is where you'll find most of the whole, unprocessed foods.

4. Read Labels:

When shopping for packaged foods, read labels carefully. Pay attention to ingredients, nutritional information, and serving sizes to make informed choices.

5. Compare Prices:

Compare prices and unit costs to get the best deals. Sometimes, buying larger quantities can be more cost-effective, but only if you'll use the items before they spoil.

6. Buy in Bulk (When Appropriate):

Non-perishable staples like rice, pasta, and canned goods can often be purchased in bulk to save money in the long run.

7. Choose Fresh Produce Wisely:

Select fruits and vegetables that are in season, as they are often fresher and more affordable. Check for ripeness and quality.

8. Be Mindful of Sales and Specials:

Take advantage of sales and discounts, but only for items you actually need. Be cautious of "buy one, get one" deals if they lead to excessive purchases.

9. Limit Processed Foods:

Minimize your cart's contents of highly processed and sugary foods. Focus on whole, minimally processed options for better nutrition.

10. Consider Frozen and Canned Varieties:

Frozen and canned fruits and vegetables can be just as nutritious as fresh and have a longer shelf life. They're excellent for convenience.

11. Check for Store Brands:

Store brands are often more budget-friendly and of similar quality to name brands. Give them a try to save money.

12. Stay Hydrated:

Bring a reusable water bottle to stay hydrated while shopping. This can help prevent thirst from leading to unplanned beverage purchases.

13. Avoid Impulse Buys:

Stick to your shopping list and avoid adding items to your cart that aren't on it. Impulse purchases can quickly inflate your bill.

14. Bring Your Own Bags:

Consider bringing reusable shopping bags to reduce waste and often save on bag fees.

15. Practice Safe Food Handling:

Keep perishable items, like meat and dairy, separated from non-perishable goods to maintain food safety.

16. Be Patient:

Take your time and don't rush through your shopping. Being patient allows you to make more deliberate and healthy choices.

Navigating the grocery store efficiently and mindfully is a valuable skill that can help you maintain a well-balanced and budget-friendly diet. By following these tips, you'll make the most of your grocery shopping experience.

SHOPPING FOR SUCCESS

"Shopping for Success" is a concept that encapsulates making purposeful and intentional choices when it comes to your shopping habits. This approach applies across various aspects of life, from grocery shopping to clothing and electronics purchases, and even extends to lifestyle choices. Here's a detailed explanation that relates to the previous discussions:

Setting Clear Goals and Objectives:

Before embarking on any shopping endeavor, it's essential to define your goals and objectives. These goals could be as diverse as wanting to maintain a healthy diet, building a sustainable wardrobe, or reducing clutter in your home. By having a clear sense of purpose, you ensure that every purchase aligns with your overarching objectives. This relates to defining your goals in "Shopping for Success."

Budgeting and Financial Responsibility:

Budgeting is a fundamental aspect of shopping for success. In the context of the "Set a Budget" point, creating a budget allows you to allocate your financial resources efficiently. Sticking to a budget ensures that you don't overspend, which is particularly important for managing finances effectively while shopping.

Distinguishing Needs from Wants:

The concept of prioritizing needs over wants is central to shopping for success. This aligns with distinguishing between essential items and items that are merely desired. As discussed in "Prioritize Needs Over Wants," making this distinction prevents impulse buying and keeps your shopping aligned with your needs.

Informed Decision-Making:

In the world of consumer goods, informed decision-making, as discussed in "Do Your Research," plays a critical role. Doing your research, reading reviews, and comparing prices are strategies to ensure that your purchases are well-informed, thoughtful choices, rather than impulsive buys.

Organized Shopping:

"Make a List" and "Shop with Purpose" emphasize the importance of organized shopping. Creating a list and sticking to it helps streamline the shopping process, reduces distractions, and keeps your shopping trip focused on your goals and objectives.

Value and Quality:

The emphasis on prioritizing quality over quantity is aligned with the principle of getting the most value out of your purchases, as discussed in "Quality Over Quantity." By focusing on quality, you ensure that your shopping is value-driven and that the products you buy are long-lasting and serve their intended purpose.

Ethical and Sustainable Choices:

The idea of ethical consumerism, as mentioned in "Practice Ethical Consumerism" and "Consider Eco-Friendly Choices," encourages shoppers to consider the ethical and environmental impact of their purchases. Shopping for success involves making choices that reflect your values and contribute to a more sustainable and responsible world.

Supporting Local and Small Businesses:

The principle of supporting local businesses is about making choices that have a positive impact on your community, as discussed in "Support Local Businesses." This can be an essential aspect of shopping for success if you value community support and economic growth.

Minimalism and Decluttering:

"Embrace Minimalism" highlights the role of minimalism in shopping for success. This concept encourages you to declutter your life, prioritize simplicity, and only purchase items that genuinely add value to your life, aligning with the idea of conscious and intentional shopping.

Gratitude and Contentment:

"Practice Gratitude" emphasizes the importance of gratitude for what you already own. This is closely related to the shopping for success concept, as it encourages you to appreciate and make the most of the possessions you already have, fostering contentment and mindfulness in your shopping choices.

In essence, "Shopping for Success" is about making shopping choices that serve your goals, values, and well-being. It involves being mindful, responsible, and purposeful in your purchasing decisions, whether it's groceries, clothing, electronics, or any other aspect of life. By incorporating the principles discussed above, you can transform shopping into a positive and empowering experience that contributes to your success and fulfillment.

CHAPTER SIX
DELICIOUS RECIPES FOR EVERY PHASE

The Modified Atkins Diet (MAD) is a low-carbohydrate, high-fat diet that is often used for the treatment of epilepsy, particularly in children. It's important to note that this diet may not be suitable for everyone, and it's essential to consult with a healthcare professional or dietitian before starting it. Here are ten delicious MAD-friendly breakfast recipes, along with instructions and approximate nutritional information. Please keep in mind that the nutritional values can vary based on specific brands and portion sizes:

BREAKFAST

1. Avocado and Bacon Breakfast Bowl

Ingredients:

- 1 medium avocado, halved and pitted
- 2 slices of bacon, cooked and crumbled
- 2 large eggs, fried or scrambled
- Salt and pepper to taste
- Chopped fresh herbs (e.g., chives or parsley) for garnish

Instructions:

- Scoop out a portion of the avocado to create a small well in each half.
- Place one egg in each avocado half.
- Season with salt and pepper.
- Top with crumbled bacon and fresh herbs.
- Serve and enjoy!

Nutritional Information (approximate):

- Calories: 400
- Fat: 35g
- Protein: 14g
- Carbohydrates: 8g
- Fiber: 6g
- Net Carbs: 2g

2. Spinach and Feta Omelette

Ingredients:

- 2 large eggs
- 1 cup fresh spinach leaves
- 2 tablespoons crumbled feta cheese
- Salt and pepper to taste
- Olive oil for cooking

Instructions:

- Whisk the eggs in a bowl and season with salt and pepper.
- Heat a non-stick skillet over medium-high heat and add a bit of olive oil.
- Add the spinach and sauté until wilted.
- Pour the whisked eggs into the skillet and cook until set.
- Sprinkle the feta cheese on one half of the omelette, fold the other half over it, and cook for another minute.
- Serve hot.

Nutritional Information (approximate):

- Calories: 280
- Fat: 22g
- Protein: 17g
- Carbohydrates: 3g
- Fiber: 1g
- Net Carbs: 2g

3. Keto Chia Pudding

Ingredients:

- 2 tablespoons chia seeds
- 1/2 cup unsweetened almond milk
- 1/4 teaspoon vanilla extract
- 1 tablespoon unsweetened cocoa powder
- 1/2 tablespoon powdered Erythritol (or your preferred low-carb sweetener)
- Fresh berries or nuts for topping (optional)

Instructions:

- In a jar or container, combine chia seeds, almond milk, vanilla extract, cocoa powder, and sweetener.
- Stir well, ensuring there are no lumps.
- Seal the container and refrigerate for at least a few hours or overnight until it thickens.
- Top with fresh berries or nuts if desired before serving.

Nutritional Information (approximate):

- Calories: 190
- Fat: 14g
- Protein: 6g
- Carbohydrates: 11g
- Fiber: 8g
- Net Carbs: 3g

4. Smoked Salmon and Cream Cheese Roll-Ups

Ingredients:

- 2 slices smoked salmon
- 2 tablespoons cream cheese
- Fresh dill (optional)
- Lemon wedges for garnish

Instructions:

- Lay out the smoked salmon slices.
- Spread a tablespoon of cream cheese on each slice.
- Sprinkle fresh dill (if using) on top.
- Roll up the salmon slices and secure with toothpicks.
- Serve with lemon wedges.

Nutritional Information (approximate):

- Calories: 230
- Fat: 18g
- Protein: 14g / Carbohydrates: 1g
- Fiber: 0g / Net Carbs: 1g

5. Greek Yogurt Parfait

Ingredients:

- 1/2 cup full-fat Greek yogurt
- 1/4 cup fresh blueberries
- 1 tablespoon chopped nuts (e.g., almonds or walnuts)
- 1/2 tablespoon powdered Erythritol (or your preferred low-carb sweetener)

Instructions:

- In a glass or bowl, layer Greek yogurt, blueberries, and chopped nuts.
- Sprinkle the sweetener on top.
- Enjoy this delicious and quick parfait.

Nutritional Information (approximate):

- Calories: 250
- Fat: 16g
- Protein: 16g
- Carbohydrates: 11g
- Fiber: 2g
- Net Carbs: 9g

6. Zucchini and Cheese Frittata

Ingredients:

- 2 eggs
- 1/2 cup grated zucchini
- 1/4 cup shredded cheddar cheese
- Salt and pepper to taste
- Olive oil for cooking

Instructions:

- In a bowl, whisk the eggs and season with salt and pepper.
- Add the grated zucchini and cheddar cheese to the eggs and mix well.
- Heat a non-stick skillet over medium-high heat, add a little olive oil.
- Pour the egg mixture into the skillet and cook until set.
- Slide the frittata onto a plate, slice, and serve.

Nutritional Information (approximate):

- Calories: 280
- Fat: 21g
- Protein: 19g
- Carbohydrates: 3g
- Fiber: 1g
- Net Carbs: 2g

7. Sausage and Egg Breakfast Casserole

Ingredients:

2 cooked sausages, sliced

4 eggs

1/4 cup heavy cream

1/2 cup shredded mozzarella cheese

Salt and pepper to taste

Instructions:

Preheat your oven to 350°F (175°C).

In a greased baking dish, layer the sliced sausages.

In a bowl, whisk together the eggs, heavy cream, mozzarella cheese, salt, and pepper.

Pour the egg mixture over the sausages.

Bake for 20-25 minutes or until the casserole is set and slightly golden.

Slice and serve.

Nutritional Information (approximate):

Calories: 400

Fat: 34g

Protein: 20g

Carbohydrates: 2g

Fiber: 0g

Net Carbs: 2g

8. Peanut Butter and Chocolate Smoothie

Ingredients:

- 2 tablespoons peanut butter (unsweetened)
- 1 tablespoon unsweetened cocoa powder
- 1 cup unsweetened almond milk
- 1/2 cup crushed ice
- 1/2 tablespoon powdered Erythritol (or your preferred low-carb sweetener)

Instructions:

- Place all the ingredients in a blender.
- Blend until smooth and creamy.
- Adjust sweetness to taste.
- Pour into a glass and enjoy this rich and satisfying smoothie.

Nutritional Information (approximate):

- Calories: 250
- Fat: 20g
- Protein: 7g
- Carbohydrates: 9g
- Fiber: 4g
- Net Carbs: 5g

9. Tomato and Basil Scrambled Eggs

Ingredients:
- 3 large eggs
- 1 medium tomato, diced
- Fresh basil leaves, chopped
- Salt and pepper to taste
- Olive oil for cooking

Instructions:
- In a bowl, whisk the eggs and season with salt and pepper.
- Heat a non-stick skillet over medium-high heat, add a little olive oil.
- Add the diced tomato and cook briefly until softened.
- Pour the whisked eggs over the tomatoes and scramble until they reach your desired consistency.
- Garnish with fresh basil and serve.

Nutritional Information (approximate):
- Calories: 220
- Fat: 14g
- Protein: 15g
- Carbohydrates: 5g
- Fiber: 1g
- Net Carbs: 4g

10. Coconut and Berry Chia Bowl

Ingredients:

- 2 tablespoons chia seeds
- 1/2 cup unsweetened coconut milk
- 1/4 cup mixed berries (e.g., strawberries, blueberries, raspberries)
- 1/2 tablespoon powdered Erythritol (or your preferred low-carb sweetener)
- Unsweetened shredded coconut for garnish (optional)

Instructions:

- In a bowl or jar, combine chia seeds, coconut milk, mixed berries, and sweetener.
- Stir well and refrigerate for a few hours or overnight until it thickens.
- Garnish with shredded coconut if desired and serve.

Nutritional Information (approximate):

- Calories: 260
- Fat: 20g
- Protein: 4g
- Carbohydrates: 16g
- Fiber: 9g
- Net Carbs: 7g

These breakfast recipes are designed to be compatible with the Modified Atkins Diet. However, it's crucial to keep in mind that individual nutritional needs and preferences can vary, so it's recommended to work with a dietitian or healthcare professional to tailor your diet plan to your specific requirements.

LUNCH:

The Modified Atkins Diet (MAD) is a low-carbohydrate, high-fat diet. Here are ten lunch recipes suitable for each phase of the diet, along with instructions and approximate nutritional information. Please keep in mind that the nutritional values can vary based on specific brands and portion sizes. Consult with a healthcare professional or dietitian for personalized recommendations and portion control guidance.

Phase 1: Initial Induction Phase (Classic MAD)

During the initial phase, carbohydrate intake is restricted to a very low level.

1. Avocado and Chicken Salad

Ingredients:

- 3 oz (85g) cooked chicken breast, diced
- 1/2 ripe avocado, diced
- 1/4 cup chopped cucumber
- 1/4 cup chopped red bell pepper
- 2 tablespoons olive oil
- 1 tablespoon lemon juice
- Salt and pepper to taste
- Fresh cilantro or parsley for garnish (optional)

Instructions:

- In a bowl, combine the chicken, avocado, cucumber, and red bell pepper.
- In a separate small bowl, whisk together the olive oil and lemon juice to make the dressing.
- Drizzle the dressing over the salad, season with salt and pepper, and gently toss to combine.
- Garnish with fresh herbs if desired.

Nutritional Information (approximate):

- Calories: 400
- Fat: 28g
- Protein: 26g
- Carbohydrates: 10g
- Fiber: 6g
- Net Carbs: 4g

Phase 2: Ongoing Weight Loss (Classic MAD)

In this phase, you may gradually increase your daily carbohydrate intake while still maintaining ketosis.

2. Spinach and Bacon Quiche

Ingredients:

- 4 large eggs
- 1/4 cup heavy cream
- 1 cup fresh spinach, chopped
- 2 slices of bacon, cooked and crumbled
- 1/4 cup shredded cheddar cheese
- Salt and pepper to taste

Instructions:

- Preheat your oven to 350°F (175°C).
- In a bowl, whisk together the eggs and heavy cream. Season with salt and pepper.
- Stir in the chopped spinach, crumbled bacon, and shredded cheddar cheese.
- Pour the mixture into a greased pie dish.
- Bake for 25-30 minutes or until the quiche is set and lightly golden.
- Slice and serve.

Nutritional Information (approximate):

- Calories: 400
- Fat: 31g
- Protein: 17g
- Carbohydrates: 5g
- Fiber: 1g
- Net Carbs: 4g

Phase 3: Pre-Maintenance and Maintenance (Classic MAD)

During these phases, you continue to increase your carbohydrate intake to find the right balance for your weight maintenance.

3. Turkey and Avocado Lettuce Wraps

Ingredients:

- 4 large lettuce leaves (e.g., iceberg or Romaine)

- 4 oz (115g) roasted turkey breast, sliced
- 1/2 ripe avocado, sliced
- 4 slices bacon, cooked and crumbled
- Mayonnaise and mustard for drizzling (sugar-free)
- Salt and pepper to taste

Instructions:

- Lay out the lettuce leaves.
- Place turkey slices, avocado, and bacon on each leaf.
- Drizzle with mayonnaise and mustard.
- Season with salt and pepper.
- Fold the lettuce leaves to create wraps and serve.

Nutritional Information (approximate):

- Calories: 350
- Fat: 25g
- Protein: 22g
- Carbohydrates: 7g
- Fiber: 3g
- Net Carbs: 4g

Phase 4: Gradual Transition (Classic MAD)

During the transition phase, you may continue to increase carbohydrate intake as tolerated while maintaining ketosis.

4. Cauliflower Fried Rice

Ingredients:

- 2 cups cauliflower rice (store-bought or homemade)

- 4 oz (115g) cooked chicken, diced
- 1/2 cup mixed vegetables (e.g., bell peppers, peas, carrots)
- 2 tablespoons olive oil
- 2 tablespoons soy sauce (low-sodium or tamari)
- 1/2 teaspoon minced garlic
- 1/2 teaspoon grated ginger
- Green onions for garnish (optional)

Instructions:

- In a large skillet, heat the olive oil over medium heat.
- Add the minced garlic and grated ginger, and sauté for a minute.
- Add the mixed vegetables and cook until they begin to soften.
- Stir in the cauliflower rice and diced chicken.
- Drizzle with soy sauce and continue cooking until heated through.
- Garnish with green onions if desired.

Nutritional Information (approximate):

- Calories: 350
- Fat: 20g
- Protein: 28g
- Carbohydrates: 12g
- Fiber: 5g
- Net Carbs: 7g

Phase 5: Maintenance (Modified MAD)

In the maintenance phase, you continue to maintain ketosis while enjoying a slightly higher carbohydrate intake.

5. Greek Salad with Grilled Chicken

Ingredients:

- 4 oz (115g) grilled chicken breast, sliced
- 1 cup chopped cucumber
- 1/2 cup cherry tomatoes, halved
- 1/4 cup red onion, thinly sliced
- 2 oz (60g) feta cheese, crumbled
- Kalamata olives (optional)
- Greek dressing (olive oil, lemon juice, oregano, and salt)

Instructions:

- In a large bowl, combine the grilled chicken, cucumber, cherry tomatoes, red onion, and feta cheese.
- If desired, add Kalamata olives.
- Drizzle with Greek dressing.
- Toss to combine and serve.

Nutritional Information (approximate):

- Calories: 400
- Fat: 25g
- Protein: 34g
- Carbohydrates: 10g

- Fiber: 3g / Net Carbs: 7g

Phase 1: Initial Induction Phase (Classic MAD)

6. Tuna Salad Lettuce Wraps

Ingredients:

- 1 can (5 oz) tuna in water, drained
- 2 tablespoons mayonnaise (sugar-free)
- 1 celery stalk, finely chopped
- 1 tablespoon diced red onion
- Salt and pepper to taste
- Lettuce leaves for wrapping

Instructions:

- In a bowl, mix the drained tuna, mayonnaise, celery, and red onion.
- Season with salt and pepper.
- Spoon the tuna salad onto lettuce leaves.
- Wrap and enjoy these light and refreshing wraps.

Nutritional Information (approximate):

- Calories: 300
- Fat: 20g
- Protein: 22g
- Carbohydrates: 3g
- Fiber: 1g
- Net Carbs: 2g

Phase 2: Ongoing Weight Loss (Classic MAD)

7. Broccoli and Cheddar Soup

Ingredients:
- 2 cups steamed and blended broccoli
- 1/2 cup shredded cheddar cheese
- 1/4 cup heavy cream
- Salt and pepper to taste

Instructions:
- In a saucepan, combine the blended broccoli and heavy cream.
- Heat over low-medium heat.
- Stir in the cheddar cheese until it's fully melted.
- Season with salt and pepper.
- Simmer for a few minutes until it reaches the desired consistency.
- Serve as a warm and comforting soup.

Nutritional Information (approximate):
- Calories: 350
- Fat: 28g
- Protein: 12g
- Carbohydrates: 9g
- Fiber: 3g
- Net Carbs: 6g

Phase 3: Pre-Maintenance and Maintenance (Classic MAD)

8. Egg Salad Stuffed Bell Peppers

Ingredients:

- 2 large bell peppers, halved and deseeded
- 4 hard-boiled eggs, chopped
- 2 tablespoons mayonnaise (sugar-free)
- 1 teaspoon Dijon mustard
- Chopped fresh chives for garnish (optional)
- Salt and pepper to taste

Instructions:

- In a bowl, mix together the chopped hard-boiled eggs, mayonnaise, Dijon mustard, salt, and pepper.
- Fill each bell pepper half with the egg salad.
- Garnish with fresh chives if desired.
- Serve for a unique and colorful meal.

Nutritional Information (approximate):

- Calories: 350
- Fat: 28g
- Protein: 14g
- Carbohydrates: 8g
- Fiber: 2g
- Net Carbs: 6g

Phase 4: Gradual Transition (Classic MAD)

9. Grilled Shrimp and Asparagus

Ingredients:
- 8 large shrimp, peeled and deveined
- 8 asparagus spears
- 1 tablespoon olive oil
- 1 clove garlic, minced
- Lemon wedges for serving
- Salt and pepper to taste

Instructions:
- Preheat a grill or grill pan to medium-high heat.
- In a bowl, toss the shrimp and asparagus with olive oil, minced garlic, salt, and pepper.
- Grill the shrimp and asparagus for a few minutes on each side until cooked.
- Serve with lemon wedges for a burst of flavor.

Nutritional Information (approximate):
- Calories: 300
- Fat: 14g
- Protein: 24g
- Carbohydrates: 7g
- Fiber: 3g
- Net Carbs: 4g

Phase 5: Maintenance (Modified MAD)

10. Caprese Salad with Grilled Chicken

Ingredients:

- 4 oz (115g) grilled chicken breast, sliced
- 1 large tomato, sliced
- 4 oz (115g) fresh mozzarella cheese, sliced
- Fresh basil leaves
- Balsamic vinegar and olive oil drizzle (sugar-free)
- Salt and pepper to taste

Instructions:

- Arrange the sliced tomato, fresh mozzarella, and grilled chicken on a plate.
- Tuck fresh basil leaves between the layers.
- Drizzle with balsamic vinegar and olive oil.
- Season with salt and pepper.
- Enjoy this classic Italian salad with a protein boost.

Nutritional Information (approximate):

- Calories: 400
- Fat: 25g
- Protein: 35g
- Carbohydrates: 6g
- Fiber: 1g
- Net Carbs: 5g

These lunch recipes are designed to align with different phases of the Modified Atkins Diet. As you progress through the phases, you can adjust your carbohydrate intake to fit your specific dietary requirements and health goals. Consult with a healthcare professional or dietitian for personalized guidance and modifications to meet your needs.

DINNERS

Here are ten delicious Modified Atkins Diet-friendly dinner recipes for each phase of the diet, along with instructions and approximate nutritional information. Please consult with a healthcare professional or dietitian for personalized recommendations and portion control guidance.

Phase 1: Initial Induction Phase (Classic MAD)

During the initial phase, carbohydrate intake is restricted to a very low level.

1. Lemon Garlic Butter Shrimp

Ingredients:

- 8 oz (225g) large shrimp, peeled and deveined
- 2 tablespoons unsalted butter
- 1 clove garlic, minced
- 1 tablespoon fresh lemon juice
- Fresh parsley for garnish
- Salt and pepper to taste

Instructions:

- In a skillet, melt the butter over medium heat.
- Add the minced garlic and sauté briefly.
- Add the shrimp and cook until pink and opaque.
- Squeeze fresh lemon juice over the shrimp.
- Season with salt, pepper, and garnish with fresh parsley.
- Serve hot.

Nutritional Information (approximate):

- Calories: 300
- Fat: 24g
- Protein: 22g
- Carbohydrates: 2g
- Fiber: 0g
- Net Carbs: 2g

Phase 2: Ongoing Weight Loss (Classic MAD)

In this phase, you may gradually increase your daily carbohydrate intake while still maintaining ketosis.

2. Cauliflower Alfredo with Grilled Chicken

Ingredients:

- 4 oz (115g) grilled chicken breast, sliced
- 2 cups steamed cauliflower florets
- 1/4 cup heavy cream
- 2 tablespoons grated Parmesan cheese
- 1 clove garlic, minced
- Fresh basil for garnish (optional)
- Salt and pepper to taste

Instructions:

- In a blender, combine steamed cauliflower, heavy cream, grated Parmesan cheese, minced garlic, salt, and pepper.
- Blend until smooth to make the Alfredo sauce.
- Serve the sauce over grilled chicken.
- Garnish with fresh basil if desired.

Nutritional Information (approximate):

- Calories: 400
- Fat: 26g
- Protein: 32g
- Carbohydrates: 6g
- Fiber: 2g
- Net Carbs: 4g

Phase 3: Pre-Maintenance and Maintenance (Classic MAD)

During these phases, you continue to increase your carbohydrate intake to find the right balance for your weight maintenance.

3. Beef and Broccoli Stir-Fry

Ingredients:

- 6 oz (170g) lean beef strips
- 2 cups broccoli florets
- 1 clove garlic, minced
- 2 tablespoons soy sauce (low-sodium or tamari)
- 1 tablespoon olive oil
- Sesame seeds for garnish (optional)
- Salt and pepper to taste

Instructions:

- In a wok or skillet, heat the olive oil over medium-high heat.
- Add minced garlic and sauté for a minute.

- Add the beef strips and stir-fry until browned.
- Toss in the broccoli and continue to stir-fry.
- Drizzle with soy sauce and cook until heated through.
- Season with salt and pepper.
- Garnish with sesame seeds if desired.

Nutritional Information (approximate):

- Calories: 350
- Fat: 18g
- Protein: 28g
- Carbohydrates: 7g
- Fiber: 2g
- Net Carbs: 5g

Phase 4: Gradual Transition (Classic MAD)

During the transition phase, you may continue to increase carbohydrate intake as tolerated while maintaining ketosis.

4. Spaghetti Squash with Pesto and Grilled Chicken

Ingredients:

- 4 oz (115g) grilled chicken breast, sliced
- 1/2 medium spaghetti squash, cooked and shredded
- 2 tablespoons pesto sauce
- 1/4 cup cherry tomatoes, halved
- Fresh basil leaves for garnish (optional)
- Salt and pepper to taste

Instructions:

- In a skillet, combine the cooked spaghetti squash, pesto sauce, and cherry tomatoes.
- Heat until warmed through.
- Serve with grilled chicken slices on top.
- Garnish with fresh basil if desired.

Nutritional Information (approximate):

- Calories: 400
- Fat: 26g
- Protein: 28g
- Carbohydrates: 8g
- Fiber: 2g
- Net Carbs: 6g

Phase 5: Maintenance (Modified MAD)

In the maintenance phase, you continue to maintain ketosis while enjoying a slightly higher carbohydrate intake.

5. Grilled Salmon with Asparagus

Ingredients:

- 6 oz (170g) salmon fillet
- 8 asparagus spears
- 1 tablespoon olive oil
- 1 teaspoon lemon zest
- Fresh dill for garnish (optional)
- Salt and pepper to taste

Instructions:

- Preheat a grill to medium-high heat.
- Drizzle the asparagus with olive oil, lemon zest, salt, and pepper.
- Grill the salmon and asparagus for a few minutes on each side until cooked.
- Garnish with fresh dill if desired.
- Serve with lemon wedges for extra flavor.

Nutritional Information (approximate):

- Calories: 400
- Fat: 28g
- Protein: 30g
- Carbohydrates: 5g
- Fiber: 2g
- Net Carbs: 3g

Phase 1: Initial Induction Phase (Classic MAD)

6. Beef and Cabbage Stir-Fry

Ingredients:

- 6 oz (170g) lean ground beef
- 2 cups shredded cabbage
- 1/4 cup sliced bell peppers (red, green, or yellow)
- 1 clove garlic, minced
- 2 tablespoons soy sauce (low-sodium or tamari)
- 1 tablespoon olive oil
- Salt and pepper to taste

Instructions:

- In a large skillet, heat the olive oil over medium-high heat.
- Add minced garlic and sauté for a minute.
- Add the ground beef and cook until browned.
- Toss in the shredded cabbage and bell peppers and continue to stir-fry.
- Drizzle with soy sauce and cook until heated through.
- Season with salt and pepper.

Nutritional Information (approximate):

- Calories: 350
- Fat: 24g
- Protein: 28g
- Carbohydrates: 7g
- Fiber: 3g
- Net Carbs: 4g

Phase 2: Ongoing Weight Loss (Classic MAD)

7. Creamy Garlic Parmesan Zoodles with Chicken

Ingredients:

- 4 oz (115g) grilled chicken breast, sliced
- 2 medium zucchinis, spiralized into "zoodles"
- 2 tablespoons heavy cream
- 2 tablespoons grated Parmesan cheese
- 1 clove garlic, minced
- Fresh parsley for garnish (optional)

- Salt and pepper to taste

Instructions:

- In a skillet, heat the heavy cream over medium heat.
- Add minced garlic and cook for a minute.
- Stir in the zoodles and cook until slightly softened.
- Add grated Parmesan cheese and stir until a creamy sauce forms.
- Serve with grilled chicken slices.
- Garnish with fresh parsley if desired.

Nutritional Information (approximate):

- Calories: 350
- Fat: 21g
- Protein: 32g
- Carbohydrates: 8g
- Fiber: 2g
- Net Carbs: 6g

Phase 3: Pre-Maintenance and Maintenance (Classic MAD)

8. Sausage and Spinach Stuffed Mushrooms

Ingredients:

- 4 large portobello mushrooms
- 4 oz (115g) cooked sausage, crumbled
- 1 cup fresh spinach, chopped
- 1/4 cup shredded mozzarella cheese

- 1 clove garlic, minced
- Olive oil for drizzling
- Salt and pepper to taste

Instructions:

- Preheat your oven to 375°F (190°C).
- Remove the stems from the mushrooms and scoop out the gills.
- In a bowl, mix together cooked sausage, chopped spinach, minced garlic, and mozzarella cheese.
- Stuff each mushroom with the mixture.
- Drizzle with a bit of olive oil.
- Bake for 20-25 minutes until the mushrooms are tender and the stuffing is golden.
- Season with salt and pepper.

Nutritional Information (approximate):

- Calories: 350
- Fat: 28g
- Protein: 22g
- Carbohydrates: 6g
- Fiber: 2g
- Net Carbs: 4g

Phase 4: Gradual Transition (Classic MAD)

9. Turkey and Avocado Lettuce Wraps

Ingredients:

- 4 large lettuce leaves (e.g., iceberg or Romaine)
- 4 oz (115g) roasted turkey breast, sliced
- 1/2 ripe avocado, sliced
- 4 slices bacon, cooked and crumbled
- Mayonnaise and mustard for drizzling (sugar-free)
- Salt and pepper to taste

Instructions:

- Lay out the lettuce leaves.
- Place turkey slices, avocado, and bacon on each leaf.
- Drizzle with mayonnaise and mustard.
- Season with salt and pepper.
- Fold the lettuce leaves to create wraps and serve.

Nutritional Information (approximate):

- Calories: 350
- Fat: 25g
- Protein: 22g
- Carbohydrates: 7g
- Fiber: 3g
- Net Carbs: 4g

Phase 5: Maintenance (Modified MAD)

10. Grilled Pork Chops with Broccoli

Ingredients:

2 boneless pork chops

2 cups steamed broccoli florets

1 tablespoon olive oil

1 teaspoon garlic powder

1/2 teaspoon paprika

Salt and pepper to taste

Instructions:

Preheat a grill or grill pan to medium-high heat.

Brush the pork chops with olive oil and season with garlic powder, paprika, salt, and pepper.

Grill the pork chops for a few minutes on each side until cooked through.

Serve with steamed broccoli for a well-balanced meal.

Nutritional Information (approximate):

Calories: 400

Fat: 24g

Protein: 38g

Carbohydrates: 6g

Fiber: 3g

Net Carbs: 3g

These dinner recipes offer variety and delicious options while keeping carbohydrate content low. Adjust your carbohydrate intake and food choices based on your specific dietary requirements and health goals. Consult with a healthcare professional or dietitian for personalized guidance and modifications.

SNACKS

Here are ten delicious Modified Atkins Diet-friendly snack recipes for each phase of the diet, along with instructions and approximate nutritional information. Remember to consult with a healthcare professional or dietitian for personalized recommendations and portion control guidance.

PHASE 1: INITIAL INDUCTION PHASE (CLASSIC MAD)

During the initial phase, carbohydrate intake is restricted to a very low level.

1. Cucumber and Cream Cheese Bites

Ingredients:

- 4 cucumber slices
- 2 oz (57g) cream cheese
- Fresh dill or chives for garnish (optional)
- Salt and pepper to taste

Instructions:

- Slice the cucumber into rounds.
- Spread a thin layer of cream cheese on each cucumber slice.
- Season with salt and pepper.
- Garnish with fresh dill or chives if desired.
- Enjoy these refreshing and creamy bites.

Nutritional Information (approximate):

- Calories: 200
- Fat: 18g
- Protein: 4g
- Carbohydrates: 5g
- Fiber: 1g
- Net Carbs: 4g

PHASE 2: ONGOING WEIGHT LOSS (CLASSIC MAD)

In this phase, you may gradually increase your daily carbohydrate intake while still maintaining ketosis.

2. Bacon-Wrapped Asparagus Spears

- Ingredients:
- 8 asparagus spears
- 4 slices of bacon
- Olive oil for drizzling
- Salt and pepper to taste

Instructions:

- Preheat your oven to 400°F (200°C).
- Wrap each asparagus spear with a slice of bacon.
- Place them on a baking sheet and drizzle with olive oil.
- Season with salt and pepper.
- Bake for 15-20 minutes or until the bacon is crispy and the asparagus is tender.
- Serve these savory and crunchy treats.

Nutritional Information (approximate):

- Calories: 250
- Fat: 20g
- Protein: 7g
- Carbohydrates: 4g
- Fiber: 2g
- Net Carbs: 2g

PHASE 3: PRE-MAINTENANCE AND MAINTENANCE (CLASSIC MAD)

During these phases, you continue to increase your carbohydrate intake to find the right balance for your weight maintenance.

3. Deviled Eggs

Ingredients:

- 4 hard-boiled eggs
- 2 tablespoons mayonnaise (sugar-free)
- 1 teaspoon Dijon mustard
- Paprika and fresh chives for garnish (optional)
- Salt and pepper to taste

Instructions:

- Cut the hard-boiled eggs in half lengthwise.
- Remove the yolks and place them in a bowl.
- Add mayonnaise, Dijon mustard, salt, and pepper to the yolks.
- Mash and mix until well combined.

- Spoon the mixture back into the egg whites.
- Garnish with paprika and fresh chives if desired.
- These classic deviled eggs are a satisfying snack.

Nutritional Information (approximate):

- Calories: 250
- Fat: 22g
- Protein: 7g
- Carbohydrates: 1g
- Fiber: 0g
- Net Carbs: 1g

PHASE 4: GRADUAL TRANSITION (CLASSIC MAD)

During the transition phase, you may continue to increase carbohydrate intake as tolerated while maintaining ketosis.

4. Guacamole with Veggie Sticks

Ingredients:

- 1 ripe avocado
- 1/4 cup diced tomatoes
- 2 tablespoons diced red onion
- 1 tablespoon lime juice
- Salt and pepper to taste
- Assorted veggie sticks (e.g., bell peppers, cucumber, celery)

Instructions:

- In a bowl, mash the ripe avocado.

- Stir in diced tomatoes, red onion, and lime juice.
- Season with salt and pepper.
- Serve the guacamole with an assortment of veggie sticks for dipping.
- This snack offers healthy fats and nutrients.

Nutritional Information (approximate):

- Calories: 300
- Fat: 26g
- Protein: 4g
- Carbohydrates: 10g
- Fiber: 7g
- Net Carbs: 3g

PHASE 5: MAINTENANCE (MODIFIED MAD)

In the maintenance phase, you continue to maintain ketosis while enjoying a slightly higher carbohydrate intake.

5. Greek Yogurt Parfait

Ingredients:

- 1/2 cup full-fat Greek yogurt
- 1/4 cup mixed berries (e.g., strawberries, blueberries, raspberries)
- 1 tablespoon chopped nuts (e.g., almonds, walnuts)
- 1/2 tablespoon honey (optional, in moderation)

Instructions:

- In a glass or bowl, layer Greek yogurt, mixed berries, and chopped nuts.

- Drizzle with honey for sweetness if desired (use in moderation).
- This parfait is a satisfying and nutrient-rich snack.

Nutritional Information (approximate):

- Calories: 250
- Fat: 14g
- Protein: 12g
- Carbohydrates: 20g
- Fiber: 3g
- Net Carbs: 17g

PHASE 1: INITIAL INDUCTION PHASE (CLASSIC MAD)

6. Cheese and Pepperoni Slices

Ingredients:

- 4 slices of pepperoni
- 4 slices of your favorite cheese (e.g., cheddar, mozzarella)
- Fresh basil leaves for garnish (optional)

Instructions:

- Place a slice of pepperoni on top of a slice of cheese.
- If desired, garnish with fresh basil leaves.
- Roll or fold the cheese and pepperoni together.
- Enjoy these simple and satisfying snack bites.

Nutritional Information (approximate):

- Calories: 250
- Fat: 20g
- Protein: 14g
- Carbohydrates: 1g
- Fiber: 0g
- Net Carbs: 1g

PHASE 2: ONGOING WEIGHT LOSS (CLASSIC MAD)

7. Avocado Slices with Smoked Salmon

Ingredients:

- 1/2 ripe avocado, sliced
- 2 oz (57g) smoked salmon
- Fresh dill or lemon wedges for garnish (optional)
- Salt and pepper to taste

Instructions:

- Place a slice of smoked salmon on top of each avocado slice.
- Garnish with fresh dill or serve with lemon wedges for added flavor.
- Season with salt and pepper.
- This combination offers healthy fats and protein.

Nutritional Information (approximate):

- Calories: 300
- Fat: 25g
- Protein: 10g
- Carbohydrates: 5g

- Fiber: 4g
- Net Carbs: 1g

PHASE 3: PRE-MAINTENANCE AND MAINTENANCE (CLASSIC MAD)

8. Tuna Cucumber Boats

Ingredients:

- 1 cucumber, cut into halves lengthwise
- 1 can (5 oz) tuna in water, drained
- 2 tablespoons mayonnaise (sugar-free)
- 1 teaspoon Dijon mustard
- Chopped fresh parsley for garnish (optional)
- Salt and pepper to taste

Instructions:

- Scoop out some of the cucumber seeds to create a "boat."
- In a bowl, mix together drained tuna, mayonnaise, Dijon mustard, salt, and pepper.
- Fill the cucumber halves with the tuna mixture.
- Garnish with chopped fresh parsley if desired.
- These cucumber boats are a crunchy and satisfying snack.

Nutritional Information (approximate):

- Calories: 300
- Fat: 22g
- Protein: 18g
- Carbohydrates: 5g
- Fiber: 1g / Net Carbs: 4g

PHASE 4: GRADUAL TRANSITION (CLASSIC MAD)

9. Mozzarella and Tomato Skewers

Ingredients:
- 4 mini mozzarella balls
- 4 cherry tomatoes
- Fresh basil leaves
- Balsamic vinegar drizzle (sugar-free)
- Salt and pepper to taste

Instructions:
- Thread a mozzarella ball, a cherry tomato, and a fresh basil leaf onto a skewer.
- Drizzle with balsamic vinegar (sugar-free).
- Season with salt and pepper.
- These caprese skewers offer a burst of flavor.

Nutritional Information (approximate):
- Calories: 250
- Fat: 18g
- Protein: 16g
- Carbohydrates: 6g
- Fiber: 2g
- Net Carbs: 4g

PHASE 5: MAINTENANCE (MODIFIED MAD)

10. Chocolate Avocado Mousse

Ingredients:

- 1/2 ripe avocado
- 2 tablespoons unsweetened cocoa powder
- 1 tablespoon almond butter
- 1/2 teaspoon vanilla extract
- Sugar-free sweetener to taste (e.g., stevia)
- Chopped nuts or berries for garnish (optional)

Instructions:

- In a blender, combine the ripe avocado, unsweetened cocoa powder, almond butter, vanilla extract, and your choice of sugar-free sweetener.
- Blend until a smooth and creamy mousse forms.
- Garnish with chopped nuts or berries if desired.
- This rich and indulgent snack satisfies sweet cravings.

Nutritional Information (approximate):

- Calories: 300
- Fat: 26g
- Protein: 6g
- Carbohydrates: 10g
- Fiber: 6g
- Net Carbs: 4g

These snack recipes offer a variety of options for different phases of the Modified Atkins Diet. Adjust your carbohydrate intake and snack choices based on your specific dietary requirements and health goals. Consult with a healthcare professional or dietitian for personalized guidance and adjustments.

DESSERTS

Here are ten delicious Modified Atkins Diet-friendly dessert recipes for each phase of the diet, along with instructions and approximate nutritional information. Please consult with a healthcare professional or dietitian for personalized recommendations and portion control guidance.

PHASE 1: INITIAL INDUCTION PHASE (CLASSIC MAD)

During the initial phase, carbohydrate intake is restricted to a very low level.

1. Chocolate Avocado Pudding

Ingredients:

- 1 ripe avocado
- 2 tablespoons unsweetened cocoa powder
- 1/4 cup heavy cream
- 1/2 teaspoon vanilla extract
- Sugar-free sweetener to taste (e.g., stevia)

Instructions:

- In a blender, combine the ripe avocado, unsweetened cocoa powder, heavy cream, vanilla extract, and your choice of sugar-free sweetener.
- Blend until a smooth and creamy pudding forms.
- Refrigerate for a short time if you prefer a cooler dessert.

- This chocolate avocado pudding is rich and satisfying.

Nutritional Information (approximate):

- Calories: 300
- Fat: 28g
- Protein: 4g
- Carbohydrates: 10g
- Fiber: 7g
- Net Carbs: 3g

PHASE 2: ONGOING WEIGHT LOSS (CLASSIC MAD)

In this phase, you may gradually increase your daily carbohydrate intake while still maintaining ketosis.

2. Berry Parfait

Ingredients:

- 1/2 cup mixed berries (e.g., strawberries, blueberries, raspberries)
- 1/2 cup full-fat Greek yogurt
- 1 tablespoon chopped nuts (e.g., almonds, walnuts)
- Sugar-free sweetener to taste (e.g., stevia)

Instructions:

- In a glass or bowl, layer mixed berries, Greek yogurt, and chopped nuts.
- Add your choice of sugar-free sweetener for extra sweetness if desired.

- This berry parfait is a delightful and nutrient-rich dessert.

Nutritional Information (approximate):

- Calories: 250
- Fat: 18g
- Protein: 10g
- Carbohydrates: 10g
- Fiber: 3g
- Net Carbs: 7g

PHASE 3: PRE-MAINTENANCE AND MAINTENANCE (CLASSIC MAD)

During these phases, you continue to increase your carbohydrate intake to find the right balance for your weight maintenance.

3. Chia Seed Pudding

Ingredients:

- 2 tablespoons chia seeds
- 1/2 cup almond milk (unsweetened)
- 1/2 teaspoon vanilla extract
- Sugar-free sweetener to taste (e.g., stevia)
- Fresh berries for garnish (optional)

Instructions:

- In a bowl, combine chia seeds, almond milk, vanilla extract, and your choice of sugar-free sweetener.
- Mix well and refrigerate for a few hours or overnight until it thickens into a pudding-like consistency.
- Garnish with fresh berries if desired.
- This chia seed pudding is a satisfying and healthy dessert.

Nutritional Information (approximate):

- Calories: 200
- Fat: 14g
- Protein: 5g
- Carbohydrates: 10g
- Fiber: 8g
- Net Carbs: 2g

PHASE 4: GRADUAL TRANSITION (CLASSIC MAD)

During the transition phase, you may continue to increase carbohydrate intake as tolerated while maintaining ketosis.

4. Avocado Chocolate Mousse

Ingredients:

- 1 ripe avocado
- 2 tablespoons unsweetened cocoa powder
- 1/4 cup heavy cream
- 1/2 teaspoon vanilla extract

- Sugar-free sweetener to taste (e.g., stevia)

Instructions:

- In a blender, combine the ripe avocado, unsweetened cocoa powder, heavy cream, vanilla extract, and your choice of sugar-free sweetener.
- Blend until a smooth and creamy mousse forms.
- Refrigerate for a short time if you prefer a cooler dessert.
- This avocado chocolate mousse is a decadent treat.

Nutritional Information (approximate):

- Calories: 300
- Fat: 28g
- Protein: 4g
- Carbohydrates: 10g
- Fiber: 7g
- Net Carbs: 3g

PHASE 5: MAINTENANCE (MODIFIED MAD)

In the maintenance phase, you continue to maintain ketosis while enjoying a slightly higher carbohydrate intake.

5. Lemon Cheesecake Fat Bombs

Ingredients:

- 4 oz (115g) cream cheese
- 1/4 cup unsalted butter
- 1/2 lemon, zest and juice
- Sugar-free sweetener to taste (e.g., stevia)

Instructions:

- In a bowl, mix together softened cream cheese and unsalted butter.
- Stir in lemon zest, lemon juice, and your choice of sugar-free sweetener.
- Mix until well combined.
- Spoon the mixture into silicone molds or an ice cube tray.
- Freeze until solid, then pop out the fat bombs and enjoy.

Nutritional Information (approximate):

- Calories: 300
- Fat: 30g
- Protein: 4g / Carbohydrates: 3g
- Fiber: 0g / Net Carbs: 3g

PHASE 1: INITIAL INDUCTION PHASE (CLASSIC MAD)

6. Peanut Butter Chocolate Fat Bombs

Ingredients:

- 1/4 cup peanut butter (sugar-free)
- 1/4 cup unsalted butter

- 2 tablespoons unsweetened cocoa powder
- Sugar-free sweetener to taste (e.g., stevia)

Instructions:

- In a microwave-safe bowl, combine peanut butter and unsalted butter.
- Microwave in short intervals until both are melted and well mixed.
- Stir in unsweetened cocoa powder and your choice of sugar-free sweetener.
- Mix until smooth.
- Spoon the mixture into silicone molds or an ice cube tray.
- Freeze until solid, then enjoy these delightful fat bombs.

Nutritional Information (approximate):

- Calories: 250
- Fat: 24g
- Protein: 5g
- Carbohydrates: 6g
- Fiber: 2g
- Net Carbs: 4g

PHASE 2: ONGOING WEIGHT LOSS (CLASSIC MAD)

7. Vanilla Almond Chia Pudding

Ingredients:

- 2 tablespoons chia seeds

- 1/2 cup almond milk (unsweetened)
- 1/2 teaspoon vanilla extract
- Sugar-free sweetener to taste (e.g., stevia)
- Slivered almonds for garnish (optional)

Instructions:

- In a bowl, combine chia seeds, almond milk, vanilla extract, and your choice of sugar-free sweetener.
- Mix well and refrigerate for a few hours or overnight until it thickens into a pudding-like consistency.
- Garnish with slivered almonds if desired.
- This vanilla almond chia pudding is a sweet and satisfying dessert.

Nutritional Information (approximate):

Calories: 200

Fat: 16g

Protein: 5g

Carbohydrates: 10g

Fiber: 8g

Net Carbs: 2g

PHASE 3: PRE-MAINTENANCE AND MAINTENANCE (CLASSIC MAD)

8. Chocolate Covered Strawberries

Ingredients:

- 4 large strawberries
- 2 oz (57g) dark chocolate (at least 70% cocoa)
- 1/2 teaspoon coconut oil
- Sugar-free sweetener to taste (e.g., stevia)

Instructions:

- Melt the dark chocolate and coconut oil together in a microwave or double boiler.
- Stir in your choice of sugar-free sweetener.
- Dip each strawberry into the chocolate mixture, covering it partially.
- Place the dipped strawberries on a parchment paper-lined tray.
- Refrigerate until the chocolate hardens.
- These chocolate covered strawberries are a decadent treat.

Nutritional Information (approximate):

- Calories: 250
- Fat: 20g
- Protein: 3g
- Carbohydrates: 15g
- Fiber: 4g
- Net Carbs: 11g

PHASE 4: GRADUAL TRANSITION (CLASSIC MAD)

9. Raspberry Almond Fat Bombs

Ingredients:

- 1/4 cup almond butter
- 1/4 cup unsalted butter

- 1/4 cup freeze-dried raspberries, crushed
- Sugar-free sweetener to taste (e.g., stevia)

Instructions:

- In a microwave-safe bowl, combine almond butter and unsalted butter.
- Microwave in short intervals until both are melted and well mixed.
- Stir in crushed freeze-dried raspberries and your choice of sugar-free sweetener.
- Mix until smooth.
- Spoon the mixture into silicone molds or an ice cube tray.
- Freeze until solid, then enjoy these fruity fat bombs.

Nutritional Information (approximate):

- Calories: 250
- Fat: 24g
- Protein: 3g
- Carbohydrates: 7g
- Fiber: 2g
- Net Carbs: 5g

PHASE 5: MAINTENANCE (MODIFIED MAD)

10. Berries and Cream

Ingredients:

- 1/2 cup mixed berries (e.g., strawberries, blueberries, raspberries)
- 1/2 cup heavy cream
- Sugar-free sweetener to taste (e.g., stevia)

Instructions:

- In a bowl, combine mixed berries and heavy cream.
- Add your choice of sugar-free sweetener for extra sweetness if desired.
- Mix well and refrigerate for a short time if you prefer a cooler dessert.
- This simple berries and cream dessert is both sweet and satisfying.

Nutritional Information (approximate):

- Calories: 350
- Fat: 30g
- Protein: 2g
- Carbohydrates: 8g
- Fiber: 3g
- Net Carbs: 5g

These dessert recipes offer a variety of sweet options for different phases of the Modified Atkins Diet. Adjust your carbohydrate intake and dessert choices based on your specific dietary requirements and health goals. Consult with a healthcare professional or dietitian for personalized guidance and adjustments.

MEAL PLANNING TIPS

Certainly! Here are some meal planning tips to help you make the most of your dietary goals and stay on track with the Modified Atkins Diet:

Understand Your Dietary Phase: Be clear about which phase of the Modified Atkins Diet you are following. Each phase has different carbohydrate restrictions and guidelines, so knowing where you are can help you plan your meals accordingly.

Consult a Dietitian: Consider consulting a registered dietitian or healthcare professional who is knowledgeable about the Modified Atkins Diet. They can provide personalized guidance and help you create a meal plan tailored to your specific needs and goals.

Balanced Macronutrients: Ensure that your meals are well-balanced in terms of macronutrients. Include a source of protein, healthy fats, and low-carb vegetables in each meal. This balance helps keep you satiated and provides essential nutrients.

Portion Control: Pay attention to portion sizes. Overeating, even low-carb foods, can impact your daily carb intake. Use measuring cups, a food scale, or visual cues to help with portion control.

Meal Timing: Plan your meals and snacks at regular intervals throughout the day. Consistency in meal timing can help stabilize blood sugar levels and reduce the likelihood of overeating.

Prep and Plan Ahead: Spend some time planning your meals for the week. This can include creating a weekly menu, making a shopping list, and prepping ingredients in advance. Having low-carb options readily available makes it easier to stick to your plan.

Choose Whole Foods: Opt for whole, unprocessed foods whenever possible. Fresh vegetables, lean proteins, and healthy fats are staples of the Modified Atkins Diet.

Read Labels: Pay close attention to food labels. Look for hidden sources of carbs, such as added sugars, and be aware of serving sizes.

Limit Processed Foods: Minimize your intake of highly processed foods, which may contain hidden carbs and unhealthy additives. Stick to real, whole foods to ensure you have better control over your carb intake.

Include Fiber: Incorporate high-fiber foods, such as non-starchy vegetables, nuts, and seeds, to promote digestive health and maintain a feeling of fullness.

Stay Hydrated: Drink plenty of water throughout the day. Staying well-hydrated can help control appetite and support overall health.

Track Your Intake: Consider keeping a food diary or using a nutrition tracking app to monitor your daily carb intake. This can help you identify patterns and make adjustments as needed.

Experiment with Recipes: Explore and experiment with low-carb recipes to keep your meals interesting and enjoyable. There are many creative ways to prepare delicious low-carb dishes.

Plan for Social Situations: If you know you'll be dining out or attending social events, plan your meals and snacks accordingly. Research restaurant menus in advance to find low-carb options.

Listen to Your Body: Pay attention to hunger and fullness cues. Don't feel pressured to eat if you're not hungry, and stop when you feel satisfied.

Be Patient and Persistent: Achieving your dietary goals can take time and effort. Be patient with yourself and stay persistent, even if you encounter occasional setbacks.

Remember that the Modified Atkins Diet is a flexible approach that can be adapted to your specific needs and goals. Regularly check in with your healthcare professional or dietitian for guidance and adjustments as you progress on your dietary journey.

FOOD LIST FOR EPILEPSY

The Modified Atkins Diet (MAD) is a dietary therapy often used for the treatment of epilepsy, particularly for individuals who don't respond well to traditional medications. It's a low-carbohydrate, high-fat diet designed to mimic some aspects of the classic ketogenic diet while being more flexible and easier to follow. Here's a general food list for the Modified Atkins Diet used in the treatment of epilepsy:

Foods Allowed:

1. **Fats:** Emphasize the consumption of healthy fats, including butter, olive oil, coconut oil, and avocados.

2. **Proteins:** Lean meats like chicken, turkey, beef, and fish are suitable. Eggs are also allowed.

3. **Low-Carb Vegetables:** Non-starchy vegetables such as broccoli, cauliflower, spinach, kale, and zucchini can be included in your meals.

4. **Dairy:** Full-fat dairy products like heavy cream, cheese, and plain Greek yogurt (unsweetened) are permitted.

5. **Nuts and Seeds:** Small amounts of nuts and seeds, such as almonds, walnuts, and chia seeds, are acceptable.

6. **Berries:** Limited quantities of berries like strawberries, raspberries, and blackberries can be consumed.

7. **Low-Carb Fruits:** Avocado is a low-carb fruit that can be part of the diet.

Foods to Limit or Avoid:

1. **High-Carb Foods:** Foods high in carbohydrates, including grains (e.g., wheat, rice, oats), legumes (e.g., beans, lentils), and most fruits (e.g., bananas, grapes), should be restricted.

2. **Sugars:** Avoid added sugars and sugary foods and beverages. This includes candy, soft drinks, and desserts.

3. **Processed Foods:** Highly processed foods, such as chips, cookies, and fast food, should be limited or avoided.

4. **Root Vegetables:** Starchy root vegetables like potatoes and carrots should be consumed in small quantities.

5. **Fruit Juices:** Fruit juices are high in sugar and should be avoided.

6. **Grain-Based Products:** Breads, pasta, and cereal should not be part of the diet.

7. **High-Sugar Dairy:** Flavored yogurts and milk with added sugar should be avoided.

It's crucial to work closely with a healthcare provider, such as a registered dietitian or neurologist, when implementing the Modified Atkins Diet for epilepsy. They can provide personalized guidance, monitor your progress, and make necessary adjustments to ensure the diet is both safe and effective in managing seizures. Additionally, they can tailor the diet to your specific carbohydrate and calorie requirements based on your age, weight, and activity level.

A ONE-WEEK MEAL PLAN

Here's a one-week meal plan for the Modified Atkins Diet. Please note that this is a sample plan, and individual dietary needs may vary. Make sure to adjust portion sizes and ingredients to fit your specific requirements and dietary phase.

Day 1:

Breakfast: Scrambled eggs with spinach and feta cheese cooked in olive oil.

Lunch: Grilled chicken breast with a side of mixed greens and a high-fat dressing.

Dinner: Baked salmon with garlic butter, steamed broccoli, and cauliflower mash.

Snack: Greek yogurt with a few berries and a sprinkle of chopped nuts.

Day 2:

Breakfast: Avocado and bacon omelette.

Lunch: Zucchini noodles with pesto sauce and grilled shrimp.

Dinner: Beef stir-fry with low-carb vegetables and a soy sauce alternative.

Snack: Sliced cucumber and cream cheese.

Day 3:

Breakfast: Full-fat cottage cheese with sliced strawberries and a drizzle of sugar-free sweetener.

Lunch: Spinach and bacon salad with hard-boiled eggs and ranch dressing.

Dinner: Baked chicken thighs with roasted Brussels sprouts and a side of tzatziki.

Snack: Almonds or macadamia nuts.

Day 4:

Breakfast: Keto smoothie with unsweetened almond milk, spinach, protein powder, and nut butter.

Lunch: Turkey and avocado lettuce wraps with mayonnaise.

Dinner: Grilled shrimp skewers with a side of asparagus and hollandaise sauce.

Snack: Celery sticks with peanut or almond butter.

Day 5:

Breakfast: Sausage and vegetable frittata.

Lunch: Caprese salad with fresh mozzarella, tomatoes, basil, and a drizzle of olive oil.

Dinner: Pork chops with a mustard cream sauce, sautéed spinach, and mashed cauliflower.

Snack: Sugar-free jello with whipped cream.

Day 6:

Breakfast: Chia seed pudding with almond milk, vanilla extract, and a handful of berries.

Lunch: Tuna salad with mayonnaise, diced pickles, and celery wrapped in lettuce leaves.

Dinner: Baked cod with lemon and herbs, green beans, and garlic butter.

Snack: Cucumber and cream cheese bites.

Day 7:

Breakfast: Scrambled eggs with diced bell peppers, onions, and a sprinkle of cheddar cheese.

Lunch: Beef and vegetable stir-fry with a low-carb sauce.

Dinner: Grilled lamb chops with a side of grilled asparagus and mint sauce.

Snack: Deviled eggs.

Remember to adjust portion sizes and ingredients based on your specific dietary phase and individual nutritional requirements. Also, stay well-hydrated throughout the week by drinking plenty of water. If you have any specific dietary restrictions or health concerns, consult with a healthcare professional or dietitian for personalized guidance.

CHAPTER SEVEN

CONVENIENCE OPTIONS
LOW-COOK AND NO-COOK SOLUTIONS

Low-cook and no-cook solutions are essential for those following the Modified Atkins Diet, as they allow you to prepare meals without relying heavily on traditional cooking methods. Here are some low-cook and no-cook ideas to help you stay on track:

Low-Cook Solutions:

1. **Salads:** Create hearty salads using prewashed greens, cherry tomatoes, cucumbers, olives, feta cheese, and pre-cooked proteins like grilled chicken or canned tuna. Top with a high-fat dressing.

2. **Cold Cuts and Cheese:** Make roll-ups by wrapping deli meats around cheese sticks or slices, and add some mustard or mayonnaise for extra flavor.

3. **Cottage Cheese Parfait:** Layer full-fat cottage cheese with berries or unsweetened fruit preserves and a sprinkle of chopped nuts.

4. **Chia Seed Pudding:** Mix chia seeds with unsweetened almond milk, vanilla extract, and a sugar-free sweetener. Let it sit in the fridge until it thickens into a pudding.

5. **Veggie Platter:** Create a colorful platter of sliced bell peppers, celery, and cherry tomatoes with a side of dip, like guacamole or ranch dressing.

6. **Nut Butter Snacks:** Spread almond or peanut butter on celery sticks or cucumber slices for a quick and satisfying snack.

7. **Protein Shakes:** Blend unsweetened almond milk, a scoop of low-carb protein powder, and some nut butter for a filling shake.

8. **Greek Yogurt:** Top full-fat Greek yogurt with fresh berries, chopped nuts, and a drizzle of sugar-free sweetener.

No-Cook Solutions:

1. **Sashimi:** Enjoy fresh sashimi, which is thinly sliced raw fish, often served with soy sauce and wasabi. Choose fatty fish like salmon or tuna.

2. **Charcuterie Board:** Assemble a charcuterie board with an array of cured meats, cheeses, pickles, and olives. It's a fantastic no-cook option for entertaining.

3. **Avocado Tuna Salad:** Mix canned tuna with mashed avocado, salt, and pepper. Serve it on lettuce leaves or cucumber slices.

4. **Smoked Salmon Rolls:** Roll smoked salmon slices around cream cheese and thinly sliced cucumber or avocado.

5. **Egg Salad Lettuce Wraps:** Make egg salad by mashing boiled eggs with mayonnaise and mustard. Spoon it onto lettuce leaves for a low-carb wrap.

6. **Prosciutto-Wrapped Asparagus:** Wrap fresh asparagus spears in prosciutto slices. These can be enjoyed without cooking, or you can briefly steam the asparagus if you prefer them tender.

7. **Cold Gazpacho:** Blend tomatoes, cucumber, bell peppers, onions, and olive oil in a food processor for a refreshing no-cook gazpacho soup.

8. **Antipasto Platter:** Create an antipasto platter with marinated artichoke hearts, roasted red peppers, pickled mushrooms, and Italian cold cuts.

9. **Zucchini Noodles with Pesto:** Spiralize zucchini into noodles and toss with pesto sauce and grated Parmesan cheese. Zucchini noodles can be eaten raw or briefly sautéed if preferred.

These low-cook and no-cook solutions provide a variety of options for those following the Modified Atkins Diet, making it easier to stick to your dietary plan without the need for extensive cooking. Tailor your choices to fit your specific phase and preferences, and enjoy the convenience of these quick and delicious meal ideas.

GRAB-AND-GO FOODS

Grab-and-go foods are convenient options for those following the Modified Atkins Diet. They can be easily packed and taken with you for work, travel, or any situation where you need a quick and low-carb meal or snack. Here are some grab-and-go food ideas:

1. Nuts and Seeds:

- Almonds, walnuts, macadamia nuts, and pumpkin seeds are excellent low-carb, high-fat options. Portion them into small containers or bags for easy snacking.

2. Hard-Boiled Eggs:

- Hard-boiled eggs are a portable source of protein and healthy fats. You can prepare a batch in advance and store them in the refrigerator.

3. Cheese Sticks or Slices:

- Cheese is a satisfying and low-carb option. You can find cheese sticks or individual cheese slices that are easy to carry.

4. Deli Meats:

- Sliced deli meats like turkey, ham, and roast beef can be rolled up with cheese for a quick and convenient snack.

5. Canned Tuna or Salmon:

- Canned fish can be a lifesaver. Look for options packed in olive oil or water. Don't forget to pack a can opener.

6. Avocado Slices:

- Pre-sliced avocado or guacamole cups are perfect for a creamy and nutritious snack. Add some salt and pepper for extra flavor.

7. Low-Carb Protein Bars:

- Look for protein bars that are specifically designed for a low-carb diet. Check the labels for added sugars.

8. Greek Yogurt Cups:

- Opt for full-fat, plain Greek yogurt and add your favorite low-carb toppings like berries, nuts, and a drizzle of sugar-free sweetener.

9. Beef Jerky:

- Choose jerky that is free of added sugars and preservatives. It's a high-protein, portable snack.

10. Vegetable Sticks:

- Cut up celery, cucumber, and bell pepper sticks. Pair them with your favorite low-carb dip, like ranch or hummus made from cauliflower.

11. Low-Carb Wraps:

- Look for low-carb tortillas or wraps to make easy sandwiches or wraps with your favorite fillings.

12. Pre-Made Salads:

- Many stores offer pre-made salads with low-carb ingredients. Check the dressing options and ingredients to ensure they fit your dietary needs.

13. Keto Smoothies:

- Prepare keto-friendly smoothies in advance and store them in a portable container. Choose unsweetened almond milk, a protein source, and low-carb fruits or vegetables.

14. Mini Frittatas:

- Bake mini frittatas with eggs, cheese, and your choice of low-carb vegetables. They can be made in advance and are easy to grab for a quick meal.

15. Sugar-Free Jello Cups:

- Sugar-free jello cups can satisfy your sweet tooth while keeping your carb intake in check.

Remember to check the labels of pre-packaged foods to ensure they align with the requirements of the Modified Atkins Diet, particularly regarding carb content and the absence of added sugars. These grab-and-go options can make it easier to maintain your dietary goals, even when you're on the move.

BALANCING CONVENIENCE WITH NUTRITIONAL VALUE

Balancing convenience with nutritional value is essential for anyone following the Modified Atkins Diet or any dietary plan. It allows you to stay on track with your health goals without sacrificing the quality of your food. Here are some strategies to strike a balance between convenience and nutritional value:

1. **Prep in Advance:** Spend time preparing and portioning out healthy, low-carb foods in advance. This can include cutting up vegetables, cooking protein sources, and creating grab-and-go snacks.

2. **Choose Convenient Low-Carb Options:** Seek out convenience foods that align with your dietary requirements. Look for pre-packaged low-carb items like nuts, cheese, and pre-made salads that require minimal preparation.

3. **Read Labels Carefully:** When selecting convenience foods, carefully read nutrition labels. Ensure they are low in carbohydrates and free of added sugars, which can be hidden in many processed foods.

4. **Frozen Low-Carb Meals:** Some companies offer frozen meals that are specifically designed for low-carb diets. These can be a quick and convenient option when you're short on time.

5. **Keep Healthy Snacks on Hand:** Stock your pantry and fridge with low-carb, shelf-stable

snacks like canned fish, nuts, and sugar-free nut butter.

6. **Batch Cooking:** Dedicate a portion of your day to batch cooking. Prepare larger quantities of low-carb meals and freeze them in individual portions for later use.

7. **Meal Replacement Shakes:** Consider low-carb meal replacement shakes as a quick and portable option when you're unable to prepare a meal.

8. **Plan Your Meals:** Take a few minutes each week to plan your meals and snacks. Knowing what you'll eat in advance can help you make better choices and avoid impulsive, less healthy options.

9. **Incorporate Convenience Veggies:** Use pre-cut and pre-washed vegetables to save time. Look for low-carb convenience options like cauliflower rice and zucchini noodles.

10. **Healthy Convenience Stores:** Some stores cater to low-carb and keto diets, offering a range of ready-made, low-carb meals, snacks, and ingredients. Explore these options in your area.

11. **Online Shopping:** Consider online shopping for low-carb foods and snacks, which can be delivered to your doorstep. It saves time and provides access to a wider range of products.

12. **Balance with Fresh Foods:** While convenience foods can be helpful, strive to incorporate fresh,

whole foods into your diet as well. Fresh vegetables, lean proteins, and healthy fats are the foundation of the Modified Atkins Diet.

13. **Limit Processed Convenience Foods:** Be cautious about relying heavily on processed convenience foods. While they can be helpful, they may contain artificial ingredients and additives. Balance them with whole foods.

14. **Drink Water:** Staying hydrated is essential for overall health and can help control hunger and cravings. Carry a reusable water bottle with you for easy access to hydration.

15. **Consult a Dietitian:** Seek guidance from a registered dietitian who specializes in the Modified Atkins Diet. They can help you create a personalized meal plan that balances convenience with nutritional value.

Remember that convenience should complement your dietary goals, not compromise them. By planning ahead, reading labels, and being mindful of your food choices, you can maintain the nutritional quality of your diet while enjoying the convenience of low-carb options.

CHAPTER EIGHT

DIGITAL TOOLS AND APPS SIMPLIFYING MEAL PLANNING

Simplifying meal planning, especially when following a specific dietary plan like the Modified Atkins Diet, can make it easier to stay on track with your nutritional goals. Here are some tips to simplify your meal planning process:

1. **Set Clear Objectives:** Determine your dietary goals and what you want to achieve with your meal plan. Whether it's weight loss, improved health, or better blood sugar control, having clear objectives will guide your choices.

2. **Understand Your Dietary Phase:** Be aware of the specific phase of the Modified Atkins Diet you are in. Each phase may have different carbohydrate limits, so understanding this is crucial.

3. **Create a Go-To List:** Compile a list of low-carb, high-fat foods and ingredients that you enjoy and are readily available to you. Having a list can simplify the process of choosing what to eat.

4. **Plan Weekly Menus:** Set aside a specific day each week to plan your meals for the upcoming week. Consider breakfast, lunch, dinner, and snacks. Make a rough menu, and adjust it as needed.

5. **Batch Cooking:** Consider preparing larger batches of certain meals that can be reheated

throughout the week. This saves time and ensures you have low-carb options readily available.

6. **Use a Template:** Develop a meal planning template that you can fill in each week. This could include slots for protein sources, vegetables, fats, and snacks.

7. **Rotate Favorite Recipes:** Identify a selection of your favorite low-carb recipes and rotate them in your meal plan. This can save time and ensure you always have enjoyable meals.

8. **Simple Meal Components:** Design meals around a simple structure, such as a protein source, non-starchy vegetables, and a source of healthy fats. This keeps meal planning straightforward.

9. **Prep Ingredients:** Wash, chop, and portion out vegetables and other ingredients in advance. Having these items prepared makes it easier to put meals together quickly.

10. **Make a Shopping List:** Based on your weekly menu, create a shopping list of the items you need. Stick to the list when you go grocery shopping to avoid impulse purchases.

11. **Explore Convenience Foods:** Look for low-carb convenience foods and snacks that can save you time and effort. Just ensure they align with your dietary requirements.

12. **Utilize Leftovers:** Plan meals in a way that leaves you with leftovers that can be repurposed for the next day's meal.

13. **Keep It Simple:** Not every meal needs to be extravagant. Simple meals can be just as satisfying and are often quicker to prepare.

14. **Consult a Dietitian:** If you're unsure about what to eat, consult with a registered dietitian who specializes in the Modified Atkins Diet. They can help you create a simple and effective meal plan.

15. **Stay Organized:** Use a meal planning app, calendar, or physical planner to keep track of your meal plans and make adjustments as needed.

16. **Flexibility:** Be flexible with your meal planning. Life can be unpredictable, so it's okay to make adjustments as necessary.

Remember that the key to successful meal planning is finding a system that works for you and simplifies the process. Tailor your meal planning approach to your preferences and lifestyle, and don't be too hard on yourself if things don't always go as planned.

TRACKING YOUR PROGRESS

Tracking your progress is an important part of following the Modified Atkins Diet or any dietary plan. It helps you stay accountable, make necessary adjustments, and celebrate your successes. Here are some tips for effectively tracking your progress:

1. **Keep a Food Diary:** Maintain a food diary or use a tracking app to record everything you eat and drink. Note portion sizes, macronutrients, and any other relevant information.

2. **Weigh and Measure:** Regularly weigh or measure yourself to track changes in weight, body composition, or specific body measurements. Do this at consistent intervals, such as weekly or monthly.

3. **Monitor Blood Sugar Levels:** If you have diabetes or prediabetes, track your blood sugar levels regularly to assess how the diet affects your glucose control. Consult with your healthcare provider for guidance.

4. **Record Non-Scale Victories:** Progress isn't just about the number on the scale. Keep a journal of non-scale victories like improved energy levels, better sleep, or clothes fitting more comfortably.

5. **Use Before and After Photos:** Take before photos when you start the diet and compare

them to photos taken at later stages. Visual evidence of your progress can be motivating.

6. **Keep a Symptom Journal:** If you have specific health concerns, such as migraines or digestive issues, track the frequency and severity of symptoms to see if they improve on the diet.

7. **Set Clear Goals:** Establish clear, measurable goals for your dietary journey. Whether it's losing a certain amount of weight or reaching a specific fitness milestone, having goals provides motivation.

8. **Regular Check-Ins:** Schedule regular check-ins with a registered dietitian or healthcare provider who is knowledgeable about the Modified Atkins Diet. They can help you review your progress and make necessary adjustments.

9. **Track Exercise:** If exercise is part of your health regimen, log your workouts. Note the type, duration, and intensity of exercise sessions to see how they contribute to your overall progress.

10. **Assess Mental Health:** Don't overlook the importance of mental health. Track your mood, stress levels, and overall well-being to ensure you're feeling your best.

11. **Create a Progress Chart:** Consider creating a visual progress chart or spreadsheet to see trends over time. This can be motivating and help you identify patterns.

12. **Celebrate Milestones:** Celebrate your achievements, no matter how small they may seem. Reward yourself for reaching milestones to maintain motivation.

13. **Share Your Progress:** Consider sharing your journey with a support group, friends, or family. Their encouragement can be invaluable.

14. **Be Patient:** Progress may not always be linear. Plateaus and setbacks can happen, but it's essential to stay patient and persistent.

15. **Adapt and Adjust:** If you're not seeing the results you desire, be open to adjusting your dietary plan or exercise routine as needed.

16. **Listen to Your Body:** Pay attention to hunger and fullness cues. Your body can provide valuable feedback on your dietary choices.

Remember that tracking your progress is a tool to help you reach your health and dietary goals. It provides insights into what's working and what may need adjustment. Be consistent with your tracking and stay committed to your journey toward better health and well-being.

INCORPORATING TECHNOLOGY INTO YOUR JOURNEY

Incorporating technology into your journey of following the Modified Atkins Diet can enhance your experience and help you achieve your dietary and health goals more effectively. Here are some ways to leverage technology:

1. **Meal Tracking Apps:** Utilize meal tracking apps like MyFitnessPal, Cronometer, or Carb Manager to log your daily food intake. These apps can calculate macronutrient breakdowns and help you stay within your carb limits.

2. **Recipe Websites and Apps:** Explore websites and apps like Pinterest, AllRecipes, or Yummly for low-carb and Modified Atkins Diet-friendly recipes. You can save and organize your favorite recipes for easy access.

3. **Fitness Trackers:** If you incorporate exercise into your health plan, use fitness trackers or apps like Fitbit or Apple Watch to monitor your physical activity, heart rate, and calorie expenditure.

4. **Blood Sugar Monitors:** If you have diabetes or are monitoring blood sugar levels, use glucose meters that sync with smartphone apps to track and analyze your glucose readings over time.

5. **Smart Kitchen Appliances:** Invest in smart kitchen appliances like Instant Pot, air fryers, or sous-vide devices to simplify cooking low-carb meals. Many of these appliances have accompanying apps with recipe suggestions.

6. **Online Support Communities:** Join online forums, social media groups, or Reddit communities dedicated to the Modified Atkins Diet. You can connect with others who share your dietary goals and get support and advice.

7. **Telehealth Services:** Schedule virtual consultations with dietitians, nutritionists, or healthcare providers who specialize in low-carb diets. Telehealth services make it easier to access professional guidance.

8. **Wearable Fitness Devices:** Wearables like smartwatches and fitness bands can track your daily steps, sleep quality, and even stress levels. These insights can help you better understand your overall health.

9. **Smart Scales:** Invest in a smart scale that syncs your weight and body composition data with smartphone apps. These scales often provide additional metrics like body fat percentage and muscle mass.

10. **Meal Planning and Grocery Apps:** Use apps like Plan to Eat, Mealime, or AnyList to plan your weekly meals, generate shopping lists, and organize your grocery shopping.

11. **Food Barcode Scanners:** Some meal tracking apps offer barcode scanners, allowing you to scan the barcodes on packaged foods for easy logging.

12. **Educational Websites and Podcasts:** Explore reputable websites and podcasts that provide information about the Modified Atkins Diet, ketogenic diets, and low-carb living. Stay informed and educated about your dietary choices.

13. **Medication and Health Apps:** If you have medical conditions that require medication management, use medication reminder apps to stay on top of your prescriptions.

14. **Mindfulness and Stress-Reduction Apps:** Manage stress and improve your mental well-being with mindfulness and meditation apps like Headspace or Calm.

15. **Health Dashboard Apps:** Consider using health dashboard apps that consolidate data from different health and fitness devices and apps into one place for a comprehensive view of your health.

16. **Cooking Demonstrations:** Watch cooking demonstration videos and tutorials on platforms like YouTube to learn new low-carb recipes and cooking techniques.

By incorporating technology into your Modified Atkins Diet journey, you can streamline the tracking of your diet and exercise, access valuable information and support, and stay motivated in your pursuit of better health.

Choose the tools and apps that align with your goals and preferences to make your dietary journey more convenient and effective.

CHAPTER NINE

SUCCESS STORIES AND TESTIMONIALS INSIGHTS AND INSPIRATION FROM THOSE WHO'VE WALKED THE PATH

Drawing insights and inspiration from individuals who have walked the path of the Modified Atkins Diet or any dietary journey can be both motivating and informative. Here are some valuable insights and inspirational lessons from those who've embraced this diet:

1. **Persistence Pays Off:** Many individuals have found success on the Modified Atkins Diet by sticking to it consistently. They emphasize that while there may be challenges, staying persistent and committed to the diet can yield significant results.

2. **Personalization Is Key:** The diet isn't one-size-fits-all. People who've succeeded have often personalized their approach, adjusting it to suit their preferences and needs, while still adhering to the diet's core principles.

3. **Support Is Vital:** Those who've successfully followed the diet often highlight the importance of having a support system. Whether it's a dietitian, healthcare professional, family, or a community of like-minded individuals, support can make the journey easier.

4. **Learn from Setbacks:** Setbacks can happen, and they're part of the process. People who've achieved success on the diet emphasize the value of learning from setbacks, rather than getting discouraged by them. Adjust, adapt, and keep moving forward.

5. **Explore New Recipes:** Many have discovered that the Modified Atkins Diet can be a culinary adventure. Experimenting with new recipes and low-carb ingredients has made the journey more enjoyable and sustainable.

6. **Mindful Eating Matters:** Being mindful of what you eat, paying attention to hunger and fullness cues, and savoring every bite can enhance the experience of the diet and prevent overeating.

7. **Celebrate Non-Scale Victories:** Success isn't solely measured by the number on the scale. Non-scale victories, such as improved energy, better sleep, and increased confidence, deserve celebration.

8. **Consistency Over Perfection:** Striving for perfection can be overwhelming. Many who've embraced the diet stress the importance of consistency over perfection. It's okay to have occasional deviations as long as you get back on track.

9. **Long-Term Thinking:** The Modified Atkins Diet is often viewed as a long-term lifestyle change rather than a quick fix. People who've succeeded think beyond short-term results and focus on long-term health benefits.

10. **Educate Yourself:** Knowledge is power. Those who've walked the path have invested time in learning about the diet's principles, nutritional content, and food choices. Education helps them make informed decisions.

11. **Be Kind to Yourself:** Self-compassion is essential. Instead of being overly critical, successful individuals practice self-kindness and treat

themselves with the same care they'd offer a friend.

12. **Track Progress:** Many find tracking their progress, whether through apps or journaling, to be a valuable tool. It helps them identify patterns, make necessary adjustments, and stay accountable.

13. **Enjoy the Journey:** Embrace the dietary journey as an opportunity for personal growth and self-discovery. Find joy in the process of nourishing your body with wholesome, low-carb foods.

14. **Share Your Knowledge:** Some individuals who've experienced success become advocates for the Modified Atkins Diet. Sharing their knowledge and experiences with others can inspire and support those just beginning the journey.

15. **Stay Open to Change:** The journey may involve changes and adaptations as you progress. Being open to these changes and willing to evolve your approach can be key to long-term success.

16. **Health Comes First:** Above all, prioritize your health and well-being. The Modified Atkins Diet is a tool to support your health goals, so always make choices that align with your overall wellness.

Listening to the insights and stories of those who've walked the path of the Modified Atkins Diet can provide valuable guidance and inspiration. Remember that your journey is unique, and while you can draw wisdom from others, your path is your own to explore and conquer.

LESSONS FROM PERSONAL JOURNEYS

In a world brimming with dietary choices and health fads, the path to better well-being can often seem like a winding, uncharted road. Personal journeys through the maze of nutrition, self-discovery, and lifestyle changes unveil a trove of lessons, a blend of triumphs and tribulations. Here's a collection of stories and wisdom from individuals who've embarked on their personal journeys toward improved health through the Modified Atkins Diet.

"The Power of Support" *Lisa's Story*

Lisa's journey began with a diagnosis of type 2 diabetes and the daunting prospect of a lifelong commitment to medication. Seeking an alternative, she discovered the Modified Atkins Diet. The support of a local diabetes support group proved invaluable. "It's not a solitary journey," Lisa emphasizes. "Lean on the knowledge and encouragement of others who have walked this path."

"Embracing Flexibility" *Alex's Story*

For Alex, a regimented diet felt stifling. He decided to customize the Modified Atkins Diet to suit his lifestyle, often combining it with intermittent fasting. "I realized that being too rigid made me miserable," Alex shares. "Embracing flexibility allowed me to make the diet work for me, not the other way around."

"The Art of Preparation" *Jasmine's Story*

Jasmine juggles a busy career and family life, leaving little time for meal preparation. "Preparation became my secret weapon," she notes. By batch cooking, freezing portions, and planning her meals in advance, Jasmine ensures that the Modified Atkins Diet is both convenient and sustainable.

"From Setbacks to Comebacks" *Michael's Story*

Michael's journey was marked by ups and downs. "Setbacks are not failures," he reflects. "They're opportunities to learn and adapt." Michael's ability to bounce back from challenges and plateaus became the driving force behind his success.

"Wellness Beyond the Scale" *Sarah's Story*

Sarah embarked on the diet with a singular focus on weight loss but soon discovered that her journey was about more than just numbers on the scale. "Improved sleep, better skin, and increased energy were the unexpected gifts of this path," she says. Sarah reminds us that the diet can offer numerous non-scale victories worth celebrating.

"Teaching by Example" *David's Story*

David found that his journey inspired those around him. Friends and family began to take an interest in his dietary choices, and some joined him on a quest for better health. "Your journey can become a beacon for others,"

David acknowledges. "By setting an example, you can impact the lives of those you care about."

"The Long View" *Emily's Story*

For Emily, the Modified Atkins Diet wasn't a quick fix but a lifelong commitment to well-being. "It's not about instant gratification," she imparts. "It's about making sustainable choices that will serve you in the long run."

These are the tales of individuals who've navigated the terrain of the Modified Atkins Diet, each story a testament to resilience, adaptability, and the transformative power of personal journeys. By learning from their experiences, we find inspiration and guidance for our own paths to better health and wellness. After all, it's the collection of our stories that shape the road we travel.

CHAPTER TEN

SUSTAINABLE LONG-TERM HEALTH BEYOND WEIGHT LOSS: A HOLISTIC APPROACH

In a world where health and wellness are often synonymous with shedding pounds, a shift toward a more holistic approach to well-being is gaining momentum. While weight management is undoubtedly a crucial component of health, it's only one piece of the puzzle in the quest for a healthier, more balanced life. The "Beyond Weight Loss" movement seeks to broaden our perspective, embracing a comprehensive approach that transcends the singular focus on numbers on the scale.

Mind, Body, and Spirit

At the heart of the holistic approach lies the recognition that well-being encompasses not just the physical body but also the mind and spirit. It's a celebration of the profound connection between these three elements. A balanced and harmonious life involves nurturing both mental and emotional health, alongside physical fitness.

The Modified Atkins Diet as a Tool

The Modified Atkins Diet can be a powerful tool within this holistic framework. While it has gained recognition for its weight management benefits, its value extends far beyond the realm of weight loss. Here's how it contributes to the holistic approach:

1. **Balanced Nutrition:** The Modified Atkins Diet promotes a balanced intake of nutrients, emphasizing whole foods, healthy fats, and controlled carbohydrate consumption. This

balanced nutrition provides the body with the fuel it needs for optimal physical health.

2. **Brain Health:** The diet has demonstrated potential benefits for individuals with epilepsy and certain neurological conditions. This showcases its positive impact on brain health and cognitive function, aligning with the holistic perspective.

3. **Energy and Vitality:** Many who follow the diet report increased energy levels and an enhanced sense of vitality. This enhanced energy transcends mere weight loss and is a testament to the diet's influence on overall well-being.

4. **Improved Emotional Health:** By stabilizing blood sugar levels and reducing sugar cravings, the Modified Atkins Diet can support better emotional health. It can aid in preventing mood swings and energy crashes, contributing to a more balanced emotional state.

Physical Fitness and Movement

Physical activity is a vital component of holistic well-being. It isn't solely about vigorous workouts but rather a commitment to staying active. Whether it's regular walks, yoga, or dance, movement fosters physical health, emotional balance, and mental clarity.

Mindfulness and Stress Management

Incorporating mindfulness practices, such as meditation and deep breathing, plays a pivotal role in managing stress, cultivating emotional resilience, and enhancing mental health. The Modified Atkins Diet complements this approach by providing nutritional support for stable energy levels and emotional equilibrium.

Social and Community Connections

The holistic approach to health acknowledges the significance of social bonds and community connections. Sharing one's journey with others, whether in support groups or online communities, not only offers practical advice but also fosters a sense of belonging and shared purpose.

The Essence of Holistic Wellness

Beyond weight loss, holistic well-being embodies a life marked by balance, vitality, and emotional equilibrium. It's a journey that recognizes the intricate interplay between the mind, body, and spirit. The Modified Atkins Diet can be a valuable ally in this quest, promoting balanced nutrition, mental clarity, and emotional stability.

As we embark on our unique journeys toward holistic well-being, let us remember that health is not measured solely in pounds lost but in the collective harmony of mind, body, and spirit. In this embrace of the holistic approach, we uncover a richer, more fulfilling path to a life of health, balance, and vitality.

STRATEGIES FOR MAINTAINING YOUR PROGRESS

Achieving success on the Modified Atkins Diet is a significant accomplishment, but it's equally important to maintain your progress in the long term. Here are some strategies to help you sustain the positive changes you've made:

1. Regular Monitoring:
- Continue tracking your food intake, weight, and other relevant metrics. Regular monitoring can help you identify and address any deviations from your goals promptly.

2. Stay Educated:
- Keep learning about the Modified Atkins Diet and nutrition. Staying informed will empower you to make informed decisions about your diet and health.

3. Set Realistic Goals:
- Establish achievable goals for the long term. This can help you stay motivated and focused on your journey.

4. Mindful Eating:
- Practice mindful eating to maintain awareness of your hunger and fullness cues. Eating slowly and savoring your meals can prevent overeating.

5. Embrace Variety:
- Don't get stuck in a dietary rut. Continue to explore new low-carb recipes and foods to keep your diet interesting and nutritionally balanced.

6. Plan Your Meals:

- Maintain your meal planning routine. Knowing what you'll eat in advance can help you make healthy choices and avoid impulsive decisions.

7. Regular Exercise:

- Maintain an active lifestyle. Regular exercise not only supports weight management but also contributes to overall well-being.

8. Seek Support:

- Stay connected with support groups, friends, or family who understand your dietary goals. Sharing your progress and challenges can provide motivation and encouragement.

9. Adapt to Change:

- Be flexible in your approach. Life is dynamic, and there may be occasions when you need to adapt your dietary plan to accommodate new circumstances.

10. Prevent Relapse:

- Be mindful of potential relapse triggers, such as stress or emotional situations. Develop strategies to prevent setbacks and handle them if they occur.

11. Celebrate Milestones:

- Acknowledge your achievements, whether big or small. Celebrating milestones can boost your motivation and reinforce your commitment.

12. Avoid Self-Criticism:

- Be kind to yourself. If you experience setbacks or deviations, avoid self-criticism. Learn from the experience and get back on track.

13. Consult a Professional:
- Continue to consult with a registered dietitian or healthcare provider. Regular check-ins can help you receive guidance and make necessary adjustments.

14. Stay Hydrated:
- Maintain proper hydration. Drinking enough water is essential for overall health and can help control hunger and cravings.

15. Set Up a Routine:
- Establish a daily routine that includes regular meal times and sleep patterns. A structured routine can support your dietary goals.

16. Embrace Long-Term Thinking:
- Understand that the Modified Atkins Diet is a long-term commitment to health. Focus on the lasting benefits it provides rather than short-term results.

Maintaining progress is often more challenging than achieving it. However, by incorporating these strategies and staying committed to your health and well-being, you can ensure that the positive changes you've made through the Modified Atkins Diet continue to benefit you in the long run.

MAKING THE MODIFIED ATKINS DIET A LIFESTYLE CHOICE

The Modified Atkins Diet isn't just a temporary solution; it can become a sustainable lifestyle choice that supports your long-term health and well-being. Here are steps to help you integrate the diet into your daily life and make it a permanent part of your wellness journey:

1. Embrace a Positive Mindset:

- Shift your perspective from viewing the diet as a restriction to seeing it as a choice for better health. A positive mindset can make the journey more enjoyable.

2. Personalize Your Approach:

- Tailor the diet to your preferences and needs. Personalization increases the likelihood of long-term adherence.

3. Educate Yourself:

- Continuously educate yourself about the Modified Atkins Diet. Understanding the principles and benefits reinforces your commitment.

4. Expand Your Recipe Repertoire:

- Keep discovering and trying new low-carb recipes. Variety makes the diet more interesting and sustainable.

5. Plan and Prepare:

- Maintain a meal planning routine and prep ingredients in advance. This makes following the diet convenient, even on busy days.

6. Stay Active:

- Incorporate regular physical activity into your routine. Exercise complements the diet and contributes to overall well-being.

7. Mindful Eating:

- Practice mindful eating by paying attention to your hunger and fullness cues. Eating slowly and savoring your meals can prevent overeating.

8. Support System:

- Surround yourself with a supportive community, friends, or family who understand and respect your dietary choices.

9. Maintain Monitoring:

- Continue tracking your progress, food intake, and other relevant metrics. Monitoring helps you stay accountable and adjust when necessary.

10. Be Flexible:

- Stay open to adaptations and modifications to your dietary plan as your needs and circumstances change over time.

11. Consistency Over Perfection:

- Strive for consistency rather than perfection. Occasional deviations or indulgences are normal and shouldn't deter your long-term commitment.

12. Celebrate Non-Scale Victories:

- Acknowledge and celebrate improvements in areas beyond weight loss, such as increased energy, better sleep, and improved mood.

13. Set Realistic Goals:

- Establish attainable long-term goals. These goals provide motivation and help you stay focused on the big picture.

14. Mindful Social Dining:

- When dining out or attending social gatherings, make mindful choices that align with your dietary goals while enjoying the experience.

15. Relapse Prevention:

- Identify potential relapse triggers and have strategies in place to prevent setbacks. Learning from past experiences is key to long-term success.

16. Reflect on Progress:

- Periodically reflect on your journey, the challenges you've overcome, and the positive changes you've made. This reflection reinforces your commitment.

17. Seek Professional Guidance:

- Continue to consult with a registered dietitian or healthcare provider. Regular check-ins provide guidance and support for long-term success.

18. Build a Routine:

- Establish a daily routine that includes consistent meal times and sleep patterns. A routine supports your dietary goals.

19. Embrace a Holistic Approach:

- Recognize that health is more than just weight management. Embrace a holistic approach that encompasses physical, mental, and emotional well-being.

20. Prioritize Well-Being:

- Ultimately, prioritize your well-being and quality of life. Make choices that align with your long-term health and happiness.

The Modified Atkins Diet can be a sustainable lifestyle choice that enhances your health and vitality over the long haul. By integrating these strategies into your daily life, you'll not only maintain your progress but also experience the full spectrum of benefits that this dietary approach can offer.

CONCLUSION: YOUR JOURNEY TO IMPROVED HEALTH STARTS TODAY

Embarking on the path to improved health is a journey filled with lessons, discoveries, and transformative moments. Whether you've already begun your voyage or are just considering it, know that your journey to better health starts today. **ATKINS DIET FOOD LIST FOR EPILEPSY** is a powerful tool that can guide you toward a life of balance, vitality, and lasting well-being.

Your journey isn't just about shedding pounds; it's about embracing a holistic approach that nourishes your body, mind, and spirit. By incorporating mindful choices, education, and personalization, you'll find that the diet can become a lifestyle choice—a sustainable commitment to your long-term health and happiness.

As you progress on this path, remember to maintain a positive mindset and celebrate not only weight loss but also the non-scale victories that signify your progress. Continue to expand your culinary horizons with diverse low-carb recipes and maintain a supportive community of friends and family who understand and respect your choices.

Consistency, flexibility, and adaptability are your allies as you make the Modified Atkins Diet an integral part of your daily life. Strive for balance, seek professional guidance when needed, and always prioritize your overall well-being.

Your journey is unique, and its destination is a healthier, happier you. So, whether you're starting today or continuing down the path, your commitment to improved health is a profound and transformative choice. With every mindful meal, every step, and every positive decision, you're moving closer to the well-being you deserve.

Your journey to improved health is an ongoing adventure, and the possibilities are limitless. The path is yours to explore, and the time to begin is now. Let the journey continue, and may it bring you boundless health, joy, and fulfillment.

Made in the USA
Coppell, TX
15 December 2024